ADVANCED
KRAV MAGA

Also by David Kahn

*Krav Maga: An Essential Guide to the
Renowned Method—for Fitness and Self-Defense*

ADVANCED
KRAV MAGA

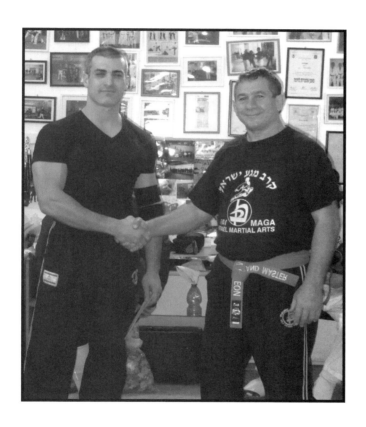

THE NEXT
LEVEL OF
FITNESS
AND
SELF-DEFENSE

DAVID KAHN

ST. MARTIN'S GRIFFIN ❧ NEW YORK

ADVANCED KRAV MAGA. Copyright © 2008 by David Kahn. All rights reserved. Printed in the United States of America. For information, address St. Martin's Press, 175 Fifth Avenue, New York, N.Y. 10010.

www.stmartins.com

Design by Susan Walsh

Interior photographs by Edward J. Greenblat

LIBRARY OF CONGRESS CATALOGING-IN-PUBLICATION DATA
Kahn, David, 1972–
    Advanced krav maga : the next level of fitness and
self-defense / David Kahn.—1st ed.
        p.   cm.
    ISBN-13: 978-0-312-36164-8
    ISBN-10: 0-312-36164-5
  1. Krav maga.   2. Self-defense.   I. Title.
    GV1111.K24   2008
    796.81—dc22
                                        2008021151

First Edition: September 2008

10 9 8 7 6 5 4 3 2 1

For my Clairety in life

In Memoriam
Instructor Dror Saporta

CONTENTS

ENDORSEMENTS

"For survival in the late 1930s, the beginning fundamentals of the *krav maga* system saved my life. This training allowed us to stand our ground and not to run. I have practiced elements of *krav maga* for over eighty years to build my reflexes, confidence, and to stay in shape."

— ERNEST KOVARY, *KRAV MAGA* STUDENT OF CREATOR IMI LICHTENFELD

"After experiencing your *krav maga*, I am compelled to write and commend your knowledge and skill of the subject and the simplicity by which you convey that knowledge. As a former Special Agent with both the United States Secret Service and the FBI, I have been through extensive training in hand-to-hand combat. I would highly recommend your teachings and the art of *krav maga* to any law enforcement entity, security professional, or individual civilian without hesitation. *Krav maga* certainly provides a solid foundation and the self-confidence to handle potentially and extremely threatening encounters. Seldom does a person have the privilege to experience the teachings of someone with your degree of knowledge, passion, and character."

— GREGORY S. SUHAJDA, FORMER SPECIAL AGENT,
UNITED STATES SECRET
SERVICE AND FBI

"I had the awesome experience, along with several other Special Agents of the Detroit FBI, of participating in a *krav maga* session with David Kahn and Rick Blitstein. The entire concept of *krav maga* is based upon simplicity. I was particularly impressed with the concept of *retzev* continuous offensive strikes, combined simultaneously with defensive moves. David has brought an already top-notch fighting system to another level, a level all law enforcement should be pursuing for the safety of its officers and the citizens."

—JOHN E. OUELLET, SPECIAL AGENT, FBI

"To my best friend and brother in arms in the fight to keep Israeli *krav maga* authentic and real, the system is grateful to have such a dedicated, skilled, loyal representative and instructor. Congratulations on the second book, *Advanced Krav Maga*, which is instrumental in helping people stay safe. I wholeheartedly recommend David Kahn's books on *krav maga* to anyone who is serious about learning how to survive today's unpredictable streets."

—N., FIRST SERGEANT AND LEAD INSTRUCTOR, ISRAEL DEFENSE FORCE
COUNTER-TERROR AND SPECIAL OPERATIONS SCHOOL

ACKNOWLEDGMENTS

I am forever grateful to Grandmaster Haim Gidon for the unique training insights and ability only he can provide as the head of the Israeli *krav maga* system and president of the Israeli Krav Maga Association (IKMA). Haim continues to develop *krav maga* at its highest level and to support the extraordinary legacy of Israeli *krav maga* creator Imi Lichtenfeld. I am indebted to my other Israeli *krav maga* instructors and close friends: Ohad, Albert, and Noam Gidon; Yoav Krayn and family; Yigal Arbiv; Eran Buaron; and Steve Moishe. Special thanks to Aldema Tzrinksky for his vital support and counsel over many years. I am grateful to my close friend N. for his strong support and the professional security expertise only he can provide. I am obliged to former *krav maga* chief military instructor Boaz Aviram, Maj. David Hasid, the IKMA board of directors, and all the IKMA members who have continued to welcome me and train with me over the years. Yet again, this book would not be possible without the expert training, support, and inspiration of *krav maga*'s backbone, the IKMA (www .kravmagaisraeli.com).

This book never would have come to be without my life-changing encounter with senior *krav maga* instructor and technical language editor Rick Blitstein. I am indebted to Rick's father, decorated World War II veteran Al Blitstein, for his recollections and insights into the development of *krav maga* in the United States beginning in 1979. I am indebted to all my *krav maga* friends, supporters, network, and affiliate instructors, including Katherina Guttman, Jerry Novack, David Ordini, Officer Mike Delahanty, Ofc. Jose Anaya, Scott Rizzo, George Foster, Thom Farrell, Dan Brown, Jason Bleitstein, Bert Witte, Rinaldo Rossi, Jonathan Levy, Steve Jansen, Asher Wilner, Ken Winokur, Rich Felsher, Sean Quinby, Elizabeth Greenman, Ethan Vogelhut, Kris Sawicki, Vitor Martin, Al Ackerman, James Sherman, Manny Sosa, Dr. Ari Malka, and, especially, senior instructor Alan Feldman, along with all those instructors about to join us. In memory of Andy Hauerstock, I would like to thank his loving family for their wonderful hospitality during my semi-annual visits to Israel. I am grateful to all our students, both in New York City and at our New Jersey–based Israeli Krav Maga United States Training Center (www.israelikrav.com). Jeff Belets and Paul Warren of Samzie's and Jim Stiles merit special thanks for their support.

I must give special thanks to senior Israeli instructor Dror Saporta and his wife, Inbar, along with my friend Bill Kingson, for helping to spearhead the necessary legal fight to preserve the name *krav maga* for all to use. Attorney David Caplan of Keats, McFarland & Wilson, LLP, is given special thanks for his legal expertise and determination to prevent the attempted trademarking of the *krav maga* name in the United States, as are Dyan Finguerra-Ducharme and Bruce Rabinovitz of Wilmer Cutler Pickering Hale and Dorr, LLP.

Thanks to A. B. Duki and Marc of the Residence Beach Hotel (www.zyvotels.com) for facilitating our semi-annual training stays in Netanya. A. J. Yolofsky and Enrique Prado merit thanks for their public support and efforts. I am also grateful to Kim and Oliver Pimley for their dedication and wonderful hospitality. I am grateful to Art Co for the sustenance to fuel my editing sessions. The Tenenbaums and Goldbergs are pillars of my life, and I cannot thank them enough. I am grateful to my colleagues at Princeton Technology Partners, especially Alan Hegedus, Ford Graham, and Kevin Davis. Emmy- and Golden Globe Award–winning actor James Gandolfini deserves special recognition and gratitude for his interest in, backing of, and support for the growth of Israeli *krav maga* as our partner in our Israeli Krav Maga United States Training Center.

A special thanks on both personal and professional levels to the Mercer County Police Academy, Somerset County Police Academy, and New Jersey State Police Academy staffs along with all of our friends and supporters in the law enforcement community, including Lieutenant Miller, Sergeant McComb, Lieutenant Maimone, Chief Emann, David Fishman, Captain Savalli (Ret.), Director Healy, Associate Director Harrison, Chief Lazzarotti, Sergeant Antonucci, Investigators Smith and Gioscio, Director Paglione, Special Agents Smith and Balceniuk, Officer Fleher, Officer Tucker, Officer Hanafee, Lieutenant Colon, Chief Ditrani, Special Agent in Charge Hammond, Special Agents Schroeder and Belle, Petty Officer First Class Alec Goenner, Special Agents Endrizal and Oulette, and former FBI and Secret Service Special Agent Suhajda along with the many other law enforcement professionals with whom we have the honor of working. Lastly, thanks to Master Gunnery Sergeant (Ret.) Cardo Urso, Major Clay Bollings, Sergeant Major (ret.) Brian Peusak, and Captain Frank Small, United States Marine Corps, for their support, and to all of our fighting men and women of the United States military and Israel Defense Forces for safeguarding our freedom.

My family has provided immeasurable support for my *krav maga* training and endeavors. Thanks to my cousins, the Rodneys, for hosting me in London for book signings and seminars. I must also thank my uncle Harry and stepfather Ed for their redoubt of support, along with my grandmother Helen. I have to thank Marvin for his superior technical support and expertise. I am also grateful to my extended family, the Browns, for their bedrock support and adding Dan to our *krav maga mishpachat*. My mother, Anne, and father, Alfred, saw the logic and the promise.

I could not have done this book and all that has come before it and will come after it without my brother and number-one friend, Abel, on his way to becoming one of the all-time great *kravists*.

Lastly, I would like to thank my good friend and expert photographer Ed Greenblat and the wonderful group at St. Martin's Press for making another book come alive along with Precision Graphics (www.precisiongraphics.com). Lisa Torri deserves special thanks. I am especially grateful to my editors, Sheila Curry Oakes and Alyse Diamond, for recognizing the need for a book on advanced *krav maga*.

FOREWORD

A teacher is judged by the quality of his student. After more than twenty-five years of teaching Israeli *krav maga*, if I am to be judged, let it be by my number-one student, David Kahn. From our chance meeting under the *sukkah* at Hillel to his first class, where I had to take him down to prove the effectiveness of *krav maga*, David has demonstrated a unique ability and desire to learn and teach *krav maga*. *Krav maga* is simple to learn for anyone, regardless of stature, gender, nationality, or age. Unfortunately, there is a need and demand for Israeli *krav maga* self-defense all over the world.

I had the honor of learning *krav maga* from its founder, first Grandmaster Imi Lichtenfeld, and I continue to learn under current Grandmaster Haim Gidon, Imi's hand-chosen successor. I lived on Kibbutz Ein Harod Me-Uchad, met Imi Lichtenfeld in 1977, and graduated from the Israeli Krav Maga Association's first international instructor's course in 1981. I grew up learning kung fu and practiced outside on the kibbutz. Some of the kibbutzniks were watching and approached me. They said, "That looks nice, but what would you do against this?" They brutalized me with chokes, bear hugs, and knife attacks—all with speed and power. I asked them, "What style is this?" They responded, "Oh, this is from the army." I found out later that these guys were in top commando units and quite adept at *krav maga*. When my commando friends took me to train, there were some older men watching. One of those men was Imi.

Many years ago I made arrangements for David to travel to *krav maga*'s source, Israel, to learn under Grandmaster Haim Gidon of the Israeli Krav Maga Association. This lineage ensures the quality of technique introduced in David's first book, *Krav Maga: An Essential Guide to the Renowned Method—for Fitness and Self-Defense* and continues with this second volume, *Advanced Krav Maga: The Next Level of Fitness and Self-Defense*. A seed does not fall far from the tree. So, by reading this book, you will be on your way to becoming a *kravist.* Enjoy.

Rick Blitstein, senior black-belt instructor

ADVANCED
KRAV MAGA

INTRODUCTION

I am proud to present *Advanced Krav Maga: The Next Level of Fitness and Self-Defense*. I would like to thank the countless readers and *krav maga* enthusiasts worldwide who contacted the Israeli Krav Maga Association and me directly following the publication of *Krav Maga: An Essential Guide to the Renowned Method—for Fitness and Self-Defense*. Israeli *krav maga* is an integral part of my life. I hope this next volume will continue to enhance and instill the Israeli fighting and self-defense method as a dynamic part of your life as well. Here, you will learn real fighting technique combined with rigorous and rewarding conditioning benefits.

The Next Level

In this volume, we continue to develop a self-defense fighting arsenal based on core yellow-, orange-, and green-belt techniques defending against unarmed attacks. These techniques derive from my translation of the Israeli Krav Maga Association (IKMA) technique guidelines. The IKMA is the governing body for Israeli *krav maga*, recognized by the Israeli government and headed by Grandmaster Haim Gidon. Grandmaster Gidon, the instructor's instructor, holds a tenth-degree black belt (red belt), the highest rank in *krav maga*. While improving the *krav maga* system daily, Haim follows founder Imi Lichtenfeld's fundamental premise that *krav maga* must work for everyone even against the most skilled adversaries. Any representation that a complete or ultimate guide to *krav maga* exists is a fallacy. Israeli *krav maga* is constantly refined and developed by Grandmaster Gidon and the IKMA professional committee. Constant improvement, evolution, and adaptability make *krav maga* a most formidable fighting system, and the genius of the system is that anyone can learn the core self-defense and fighting principles.

While space and text restraints do not allow us to illustrate the all-important *retzev*, or continuous combat follow-through, we have taken a few techniques and developed partial *retzev* to provide you with a more comprehensive insight into combined defense and attack through continuous combat motion, the heart of the Israeli *krav maga* system (the term *krav maga* means "contact combat"). The following tables serve as a summary and reference for the Israeli *krav maga* system's philosophy, tactics, and strategy.

THE *KRAV MAGA* SIX PILLARS TACTICAL GRID

Simultaneous Defense and Attack Combine your defense and offense into one complete strategy.	**Focus on Vulnerable Soft Tissue** Counterattack the vulnerable areas of your opponent's body, including the groin, eyes, and throat.
***Retzev* (Continuous Combat Motion)** Move fast, continuously, seamlessly, and determinedly, giving the attacker no time to react.	**A Building-Block Learning Process** Learn one elemental technique at a time and then build on it.
Decisive Action Be both decisive and quick in responding to a violent encounter. Do whatever is necessary to overcome a dangerous threat.	**Subduing Techniques** If possible, use subduing techniques to de-escalate a situation quickly.

THE *KRAV MAGA* MENTAL PREPARATION GRID

The Mind of a *Kravist*

In a physical confrontation, you are likely to experience a combined surge of stress, fear, and excitement. Mental and physical conditioning will allow you to harness your adrenaline and channel it into action. Mental confidence and toughness provide a decisive advantage in a violent encounter. Hone both your mental and physical skills so that you can spring into action without thinking. Only proper training can trigger this fighting response.

The Four Steps to Action

When confronted, the mind goes through a series of steps to choose a response:

1. Threat recognition
2. Situation analysis
3. Choice of action
4. Action or inaction

Reacting to an Attack

A surprise attack will force you to react from an unprepared state. Therefore, your self-defense reaction must be instinctive and reflexive. *Krav maga* training prepares you for just that. The subconscious mind turns trained responses into instinctive, immediate action.

Understanding the Human Body

The body can withstand a high amount of physical punishment. Adrenaline is a powerful energizer and allows the body to momentarily insulate itself against pain. The body's resilience works for both victim and assailant. To stop an assailant, target the body's vulnerable and vital areas using *retzev*.

THE *KRAV MAGA* MENTAL PREPARATION GRID

Making the Training as Real as Possible

Training will help you overcome the fight paralysis that can easily set in. You will learn how to alleviate fear, panic, and other sensations. You will learn effective physical techniques while mentally adjusting to a harsh, violent reality.

Visualization and Scenario Planning

Use your mind to train your body to automatically and instinctively react to danger. Visualization and scenario planning boost your confidence, reduce fear, improve your fighting technique, and help you cope with unanticipated hostile situations because you will have envisioned them beforehand.

I hope you enjoy reading this volume as much as I enjoyed writing it. Remember, train hard and be safe.

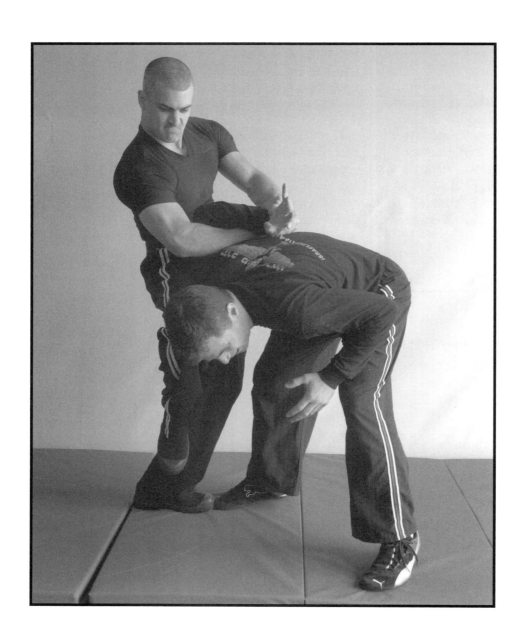

CHAPTER 1

The Israeli *Krav Maga* Advantage

The Israeli *krav maga* fighting system is designed to work against any attacker. The key is your mind-set. As my good friend N., lead counterterror instructor for the Israel Defense Forces, explains so well, you must be able to transition from a highly disadvantageous "negative five" position to an advantageous "positive five" position instinctively and instantaneously. You must turn the table on your opponent(s) immediately. Self-preservation is a powerful motivator, and so is protecting others. If you must defend yourself, you need to dominate your attacker and incapacitate him. *Krav maga*'s core techniques provide cumulative building blocks for a formidable self-defense foundation. A few mastered techniques go a long way and are highly effective in most situations.

The essence of *krav maga* is to neutralize an opponent quickly. There are no rules in an unscripted fight. This lack of rules distinguishes self-defense from sport fighting. In a sport fight the following are generally prohibited: eye gouges; throat strikes; head butts; biting; hair pulling; clawing, pinching, or twisting of the flesh; striking the spine and the back of the head; striking with the tip of the elbow; small-joint manipulation; kidney and liver strikes; clavicle strikes; kneeing or kicking the head of an opponent on the ground; and slamming an opponent to the ground on his head. These are precisely the core tactics we emphasize in *krav maga*. Keep in mind, however, that the level of force you use to defend yourself should be commensurate with the threat.

You need not master hundreds of techniques to become a *kravist*, or competent *krav maga* fighter. In *krav maga*, we prepare for any type and number of attacks. Nonviolent conflict resolution is always your best solution. While there are no set solutions for ending a fight, there are preferred methods using *retzev* (continuous combat motion) to prevail. Combined with simultaneous attack and defense, *retzev* is a seamless, decisive, and overwhelming counterattack forming the backbone of the Israeli fighting system. *Retzev* can be understood as using combined upper- and lower-body combatives, locks, chokes, throws, takedowns, and weapons interchangeably, without pause. An example might be initiating a left front kick followed immediately (prior to the left foot touching down) by a left punch, followed by a right punch, followed by a right knee, followed by a right horizontal elbow, followed by a left horizontal elbow, et cetera.

My close friend and senior IKMA instructor Rick Blitstein has some indispensable wisdom regarding conflict evolution and resolution. Rick told me of the countless times he has been confronted by larger and more physically imposing opponents and how his demeanor has helped him immeasurably. In a professional or personal capacity, your comportment says much about you, and your demeanor can end a fight before it begins.

Having the ability to walk away from confrontation is a test of discipline and moral fiber. However, you should walk away with a heightened sense of awareness while also being prepared to spring into action. Disengaging is intelligent and pragmatic for a myriad of reasons, including avoiding potential injury to you, your family, and your friends, not to mention potential criminal and civil liability.

Grandmaster Haim Gidon, head of the Israeli *krav maga* system, enforces this wisdom of de-escalation. He and his senior instructors have the same mind-set. They are the most skilled *kravists* in the world and will not suffer bullying or aggressive behavior, yet they are reticent to use their unparalleled fighting skills unless there is no other option. *Krav maga* creator Imi Lichtenfeld emphasized that you should fight only when necessary, but if fighting is necessary, end the fight quickly and decisively on your terms.

By using common sense, taking basic precautions, and presenting a confident manner, you can minimize your chances of being attacked. To prevent being caught completely off guard, you must accept the possibility of violence. Your life and well-being are not worth trading for any possessions. If someone is threatening you, especially with a weapon or if you are clearly outnumbered, comply with his demands if you can. If you cannot comply, reasoning has failed, and there is no escape, take the fight to your opponent to neutralize him. Maintaining an overall strategy to end your opponent's ability to fight is paramount.

Krav Maga Tactical Thinking

Fight positioning determines your tactical advantage. Optimally, a *kravist*—a skilled *krav maga* fighter—will move quickly to a superior and dominant position relative to his opponent, known in *krav maga* parlance as the dead side. The dead side often provides you with a decisive tactical advantage. This strategy should revolve around your capabilities and preferred tactics involving long-, medium-, and short-range combatives combined with evasive maneuvers. Positioning becomes even more important when facing multiple opponents. Once you have achieved a superior position, the opponent will have minimal ability to defend against or counter your *retzev* attack. Remember that *retzev*, which uses all parts of your body and incorporates all facets of a fight, provides an overwhelming counterattack.

Footwork and body positioning, whether standing or prone, allow you to simultaneously defend and attack, leading to the seamless combative transitions essential to *retzev*. The key to evasion is moving out of the "line of fire"—the path of an opponent's offensive combatives. Clearly, positioning yourself where you can counterattack your opponent more easily than he can attack you is most advantageous.

Fights involve different phases that are best categorized by the distance or proximity opponents maintain as the fight progresses. At long or medium range, fighters have unhindered movement to batter one another, usually involving long kicks, medium punches, and other hand strikes. At short range, knees, elbows, head butts, and biting become options. This includes a variety of standing entanglements involving medium and short strikes, trapping, clinching, throws, takedowns, and standing joint locks combined for close *retzev*. The final ground phase occurs when both fighters lock up to unbalance each other to the ground involving medium- and short-range combatives combined with locks and chokes.

Movement on the ground is different from standing movement. The nature of ground fighting can allow one opponent superior control and positioning, since the other opponent cannot run or evade as he might while standing. *Krav maga* groundwork is best defined as "what we do up, we do down" with additional specific ground-fighting capabilities. We employ many of our standing combatives on the ground, including groin, eye, and throat strikes in combination with joint breaks and dislocations designed to maim your opponent.

Breaking Your Opponent's Body

Developed as a military fighting discipline, *krav maga* employs lethal force techniques. Imi was adamant that these techniques be taught only to the military and professional security organizations. Senior IKMA instructor Rick Blitstein remembers Imi saying, "Only two people could use these techniques: a commando or a criminal." Obviously, criminals have no place in *krav maga*. Therefore, while these techniques are integrated at the highest levels of the IKMA curriculum, they are omitted from this book.

Forging an awareness of your own personal weapons (hands, forearms, elbows, knees, shins, feet, and head) and an opponent's vulnerabilities is essential to fight strategy and tactics. The human body is amazingly resilient, even when subjected to tremendous physical abuse. Pain may stop some attackers, but other individuals have very high pain thresholds. Therefore, an opponent may be stopped only when his offensive capabilities are put out of commission by joint dislocations, bone breaks, or cutting off the oxygen/blood supply to the brain, resulting in unconsciousness.

In both standing and ground fights, it becomes difficult for an opponent to fight effectively if his hands are broken. Breaking an opponent's fingers is an efficient tactic and strategy, especially against an opponent favoring pugilistic hand attacks and submission holds. Breaking larger joints and bones escalates the damage. Rendering an opponent unconscious quickly ends a fight.

Your attacker faces serious consequences if you dislocate or break a joint. The larger the joint, the more serious the consequences are to your opponent. Think about the difference between a dislocated or broken finger and a dislocated or broken elbow. Damaging a knee is also a highly effective method of incapacitating your opponent. Accordingly, the larger the joint the more difficult it will be to control and break. All joint lock dislocations and breaks are based on the biomechanical principle that bending a joint beyond its natural range of extension will damage the joint. For example, understanding the elbow or knee as a fulcrum allows many arm bar or knee bar modalities. The same is true of cervical or spine lock breaks. While the human body has around two hundred joints, we will focus on five major areas of the body for counterattack: the neck, shoulder, elbow, knee, and ankle.

A joint is at its weakest when at full extension. For example, the straight arm bar is the most direct and pragmatic arm bar. It serves as great example to examine a joint lock, when a joint is forced beyond its natural range of motion or opposite to its natural range of motion. This arm bar can be applied from a variety of body positions and angles. Ideally, you will catch your opponent with his arm already fully extended. The action mechanism involved in an arm bar (and other joint lock breaks) is to force the arm beyond its normal range of motion, damaging the elbow's structural integrity, including the joint, ligaments, and muscles. Strong breaking pressure on the back of the elbow forces the humerus forward and the ulna backward, dislocating the elbow. The wrist area provides the leverage point for breaking pressure, following a basic tenet of physics that the longer the lever, the more superior the biomechanical advantage.

Every type of lock requires moving the joint against its natural articulation, utilizing breaking pressure. While we teach certain core arm dislocation positions, once you have an understanding of the biomechanics you can apply the principles to a myriad of situations. This is especially important for the fluidity of a fight. Optimally, you will use the entire force and weight of your body to apply pressure against an opponent's joint. This is the key principle to joint locks. Two IKMA female instructors, Katherina Guttman and Elizabeth Greenman, consistently lock out skeptical students and muscular weight lifters. These *krav maga* converts come away marveling at the effectiveness of Israeli ground fighting.

If necessary, *krav maga* also employs chokes and "blood"

chokes to render an opponent unconscious or worse. With proper body positioning, you can pummel an adversary on the ground severely, with his having little defensive recourse. Movement on the ground is a skill that can be honed to a high level. Remember that whether you are standing, clinched, or on the ground, *krav maga* is designed for everyone, and a smaller opponent can defeat a larger, stronger, and perhaps more athletic one. A well-trained *kravist* will possess core training in all three combat phases. In this fighting chess game, the best way to defend against an offensive technique is to know the offensive technique. Having an array of techniques at your disposal solidifies your ability.

The Language of Krav Maga

Throughout *Advanced Krav Maga,* the following terms will appear frequently. Once you understand the language of *krav maga,* you can better understand the method.

Combative: Any manner of strike, takedown, throw, joint lock, choke, or other offensive fighting movement.

Retzev: A Hebrew word that refers to continuous motion in combat. *Retzev,* the backbone of modern Israeli *krav maga,* teaches you to move your body instinctively in combat motion without thinking about your next move. When in a dangerous situation, you'll automatically call upon your physical and mental training to launch a seamless, overwhelming counterattack using strikes, takedowns, throws, joint locks, chokes, or other offensive actions combined with evasive action. *Retzev* is quick and decisive movement merging all aspects of your *krav maga* training. Defensive movements transition automatically into offensive movements to neutralize the attack, affording your opponent little time to react.

Left outlet stance: Blades your body by turning your feet approximately 30 degrees to your right, with your left arm and left leg forward. (You can also turn 30 degrees to your left to come into a right outlet stance, with your right leg and arm forward.) You are resting on the ball of your rear foot in a comfortable and balanced position. Your feet should be parallel, with about 55 percent of your weight distributed over your front leg. Your arms are positioned in front of your face and bent slightly forward at approximately a 60-degree angle between your forearms and your upper arms. From this stance, you will move forward, laterally, and backward, moving your feet in concert.

Live side: When you are facing the front of your opponent and your opponent can see you and use both arms and both legs against you, you are facing his or her live side.

Dead side: Your opponent's dead side, in contrast to his live side, places you behind his near shoulder or facing his back. You are in an advantageous position to counterattack and control him because it is difficult for him to use his arm and leg farthest away from you to attack you. You should always move to the dead side when possible. This also places the opponent between you and any additional third-party threat.

Same side: Your same-side arm or leg faces your opponent when you are positioned opposite one another. For example, if you are directly facing your opponent and your right side is opposite your opponent's left side, your same-side arm is your right arm (opposite his left arm).

Near side: Your opponent's limb closest to your torso.

Outside defense: An outside defense counters an outside attack, that is, an attack directed at you from the outside of your body to the inside. A slap to the face and a hook punch are examples of outside attacks.

Inside defense: An inside defense defends against an inside or straight attack. This type of attack involves a thrusting motion such as jabbing your finger into someone's eye or punching someone in the nose.

Gunt: A deflection or absorption of an incoming strike by bending your elbow to touch your bicep to your forearm. The angle of deflection depends on the strike. For example, to defend against a hook punch or roundhouse kick to the head, you will position the elbow to cover your head, with the back of your arm parallel to the ground and the elbow tip facing slightly outward. The gunt may also be used to defend against knee attacks by jamming the opponent's knee with the tip of the elbow.

Glicha: A sliding movement on the balls of your feet to carry your entire body weight forward and through a combative strike to maximize its impact.

Secoul: A larger step than *glicha*, covering more distance, to carry your entire body weight forward and through a combative strike to maximize its impact.

Off angle: An attack angle that is not face-to-face.

Stepping off the line: Using footwork and body movement to take evasive action against a linear attack such as a straight punch or kick. Such movement is also referred to as **breaking the angle of attack.**

Tsai-bake: A 180-degree or semicircle step by rotating one leg back to create torque on a joint to complete a takedown or control hold.

Cavalier: A wrist takedown involving forcing an adversary's wrist to move against its natural range of motion, usually combined with *tsai-bake* for added power.

Trapping: Occurs when you pin or grab the opponent's arms with one arm, leaving you with a free arm to continue combatives.

Figure four: A control hold securing an opponent's arm, torso, or ankle to exert pressure. The control hold is enabled by using both of your arms on the joint of the wrist, shoulder, or tendon of an opponent. For example, you have secured your opponent's right wrist (his elbow is pointed toward the ground) with your right hand placed on the flat of his right hand, bending his wrist inward, with his elbow (tip toward the ground) pinned to your chest while you simultaneously slip your other arm over the top of his forearm to interlock with his arm and grab your own forearm. This positional arm control may also be used to attack the Achilles tendon with the blade of your forearm or control an opponent's torso from the rearmount. A figure four may also be applied to an opponent's torso by hooking one leg across the torso and securing it in the crook of the other leg's knee.

Mount: A formidable fighting and control position where you are straddling your opponent with his back to the ground and your heels are hooked underneath his rib cage.

Rear mount: The most advantageous control position on the ground, where you are behind and straddling your opponent (who may be faceup or facedown) with your legs wrapped (not crossed) around his midsection.

Side mount: A strong control position (example is to your opponent's right) with your right knee pressed to your opponent's hip and left knee in line with your opponent's head. The elbow closest to your opponent's head should be positioned on your opponent's ear. There are different options for hand placement, including through the opponent's legs for groin strikes and torso control.

Knee on stomach: Another strong control position, placing your full weight on your opponent's midsection and hooking your foot into your opponent's hip while resting on the ball of your foot to create a stable striking platform and wear down your opponent's body.

Side control: Your opponent is on his back and you are sitting up with your legs splayed wide and your arm controlling his head and possibly his arm closest to you.

High closed guard: Your back is to the ground with your opponent pincered between your legs, which are hooked at the ankles.

Kicking pad: A large foam shield designed to be held by a training partner for kicks and knee strikes. (See Resources for recommended products.)

Hand pad or *muy thai* pad: A maneuverable foam pad designed to be held by a training partner for punches, elbows, and other upper-body strikes. (See Resources for recommended products.)

Kravist: A term coined in *Krav Maga: An Essential Guide to the Renowned Method—for Fitness and Self-Defense* to describe a smart and prepared *krav maga* fighter.

More About Grandmaster Haim Gidon

Grandmaster Haim Gidon was *krav maga* founder Imi Lichtenfeld's top student for twenty-eight years. In 1996, Imi publicly nominated Haim as his successor. Imi remained a fixture in Haim's 21 Ben Zion Gym until his final days, sharing what he loved best with Haim— instructing, watching, and encouraging the development of the Israeli *krav maga* system. Haim continues Imi's extraordinary legacy of developing and improving Israeli *krav maga*. With each visit to Haim's gym I marvel at the improvements and additions made to the system—true to Imi's goal of creating the most modern and comprehensive self-defense and hand-to-hand fighting system in the world. Under Grandmaster Gidon's supervision and authority, the IKMA's belt guidelines (white, yellow, orange, green, blue, brown, and black 1–5 *dans*) are constantly updated. Haim has taught and molded a whole new generation of instructors and students both in Israel and abroad. Haim's unparalleled skills and those of his top students, including his sons Ohad and Noam, Yoav Krayn, Yigal Arbiv, Steve Moishe, and others, are requested worldwide by elite military units, law enforcement agencies, and civilians. Grandmaster Gidon runs annual instructor certification and advanced training courses in Israel and at the Israeli Krav Maga United States Training Center. For more information, see www.israelikrav.com and www.krav magaisraeli.com.

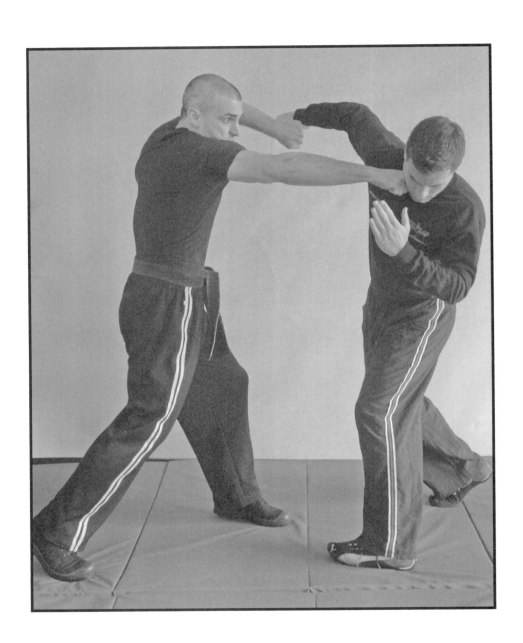

CHAPTER 2

Imi Lichtenfeld's Oldest Living Student from Bratislava

True *Kravist* Ernest Kovary

Israeli *krav maga* was designed to save lives. When Martin Knovzen walked into my *krav maga* class in Manhattan to learn the self-defense method, he told me he knew someone he thought I should meet, a man whose life was saved by *krav maga* training as World War II was erupting. Ernest Kovary began training with *krav maga* founder Imi Lichtenfeld in 1925 and was one of Imi's star pupils. I was honored to meet Ernest, a man of great learning, courage, and resounding kindness, and I must thank him again for sharing in a series of interviews his remarkable story and his unique insights into *krav maga*'s earliest stages of development.

Ernest Kovary was born in Bratislava on April 2, 1919. Ernest's grandfather had emigrated to Baltimore, Maryland, in 1891, but returned to Hungary with Ernest's American-born father. Ernest was six years old when he met fifteen-year-old Imi in the Maccabi organization, a sports club for young Jewish athletes. Before World War II, Bratislava was home to 120,000 Jews, including Imi Lichtenfeld. Imi, Ernest noted, was very active in the Maccabi organization and an ardent Zionist. Ernest recalled that Imi was an excellent gymnast, and mused, "The girls loved Imi and he loved them back. Had Imi not had so many female admirers, he would have been a world champion in everything!" Ernest remembers Imi as extremely friendly but equally tough.

Imi enjoyed performing demonstrations with Ernest by lifting Ernest over his head. Their specialty was Imi holding Ernest aloft in different acrobatic positions. "Imi liked to show me off," Ernest recalled. At age twelve, Ernest began Greco-Roman wrestling under Imi's expert coaching. Ernest observed that Imi loved to teach and coach. In sports competition, Maccabi members continued to make their mark in Slovakia. In a large regional tournament, Maccabi prevailed over five other wrestling clubs. Ernest emphasized that Imi's athletic prowess and fighting spirit stood out. The other clubs did not like that a Jewish organization won. Ernest concluded with satisfaction, "They had to respect us; we won."

Increasing anti-Semitic violence in the 1930s began to change the way Imi approached sports training. Ernest recalled that prior to 1933, anti-Semitic outbursts were isolated incidents. After 1933, the situation became progressively worse. In 1934, Ernest and his older brother, Tibor, were forced to drop out of their *gymnasium*, or high school. The year 1938 marked a turning point for Jews as violence became acute and Ernest's local *yeshiva*, or religious school, was attacked. Ernest recalled, "We mustered as many men and boys as we could to defend it."

More and more Jews became victims of bigotry and violence.

"The general attitude was that Jews would run rather than fight," noted Ernest. The Maccabi sports organization began to serve another purpose: clandestine self-defense training. The strict rules of Greco-Roman wrestling would have to be discarded. "We realized we could not follow rules if we wanted to protect ourselves," Ernest observed solemnly. "There could be no rules on the street. That would be the only way we could win." Imi developed his self-defense system accordingly. "Imi said to us that if we must break the attacker's neck to survive, that is what we will do. We needed techniques that went beyond the rules. This was the beginning of *krav maga*. Imi modified Greco-Roman wrestling, boxing, and judo and everything else in his own style." Ernest explained that the most powerful wrestlers were "heavy, slow-moving guys." Imi was "not heavy but unbelievably quick," and he "relied on his technique to win." In addition, members of the community who wanted to make *aliya*, or emigrate to British-mandate Palestine, needed self-defense training.

Ernest recalled the day World War II began: "War broke out on Friday, September 1, 1939. Slovakia was a puppet government. We had Hitler Youth in town. Next to our apartment was a small synagogue. We left the radio on and listened all evening. We woke up early the next morning to attend *shabbat* [Jewish Sabbath] services. We heard Hermann Goering say that he would not touch a hair on the head of a Jew. My father, Olivio, walked out of the building before us. He saw two Hitler Youth savagely beating Heller, our local baker, bloody, with others looking on. My father could not intervene, as he was alone. He told my brother and me not to go out.

"By 10:00 a.m., my brother and I were restless. We wondered if the attack on our baker was an isolated case or part of the larger picture. We had a large lobby in our apartment building. We peeked out of the lobby and saw the two Hitler Youths whom my father had described attacking our baker. We were not sure if they spotted us. We hurried back inside. My brother began to make his way up the steps as I followed. I heard a noise behind me. The Hitler Youth were behind us. They liked to surprise you, to attack when you were not looking. They had metal studs on their boots that they liked to stomp on you with. One of the Nazis wryly asked me, 'Are you Aryan?'

"The Hitler Youth knew we were dressed for *shabbat* services. He had something in his right hand. I don't know what he had, but he was going to try to hurt me with it. I knew they were out for blood. We could not run away. I wrote with my right hand but favored my left hand for punching. I hit him so hard with my left just below the eye that I opened up his face. His blood went everywhere, all over me. My brother had come down to see what was happening, only to be confronted by the other Nazi. Tibor wasted no time and began bludgeoning the other Hitler Youth with his hands. My brother, using our mother tongue, Esperanto, called my father for help from our upstairs apartment.

"As the second Nazi tried to escape, Tibor caught him and continued to beat him as my brother kicked him out of the door. Two street cleaners saw how my brother was beating the hell out of the other Nazi and intervened to make Tibor stop. My father had run out and had grabbed a wooden ski from our storage space. After I hit the first Nazi he still tried to come at me. We had learned from Imi's training to continue the fight until the attacker was no longer a threat. I knew I had better not kill this Nazi, but I also knew I needed to control him. I put him in a tight standing headlock. My father took the ski and hit him repeatedly over the head with it. We knew the Gestapo [German secret police] were only two blocks away. I knew the bloody sports coat would give me away, and ran up the stairs to our apartment to take off the jacket. We all went back to our apartment and locked the door.

"Word of what happened was out on the street by now. The Slovak police came with a Gestapo man in civilian clothes. The Slovak police took us into protective custody. They wanted us alive to be charged. We were brought to the police station.

Germans were running around the Slovak police station with re-volvers drawn. From the police station I could see probably more than one hundred uniformed Nazis assembling.

"Sometime later, the two Hitler Youth we beat up went to the hospital and were brought back stitched up, with casts on their broken bones. One of the Germans wanted to know the story, the real truth how they ended up so beaten up. The *Gauleiter* [Nazi district leader] heard of what happened and called the po-lice station. One of the Nazis we beat up began to tell the story, but a third German who had not been there quickly intervened to say he would tell the story [see article]. But I was present, so the third German told the *Gauleiter* he could not tell him about the incident right then. Obviously, the truth about two Jews beating up two Nazi bullies was not something they wanted out for public consumption."

Nazi propaganda presented the Kovary family's self-defense ac-tions in a twisted and diabolical light, true to the venom and falsehoods of the time. The following account of Ernest's fight was published in the German-language daily Nazi newspaper *Grenzbote*:*

OUTRAGEOUS JEWISH PROVOCATION OF IMPUDENT
ATTACK ON FS MEN [NAZIS] THE JEWISH
UNDERGROUND MUST BE LIQUIDATED

By the reporter of the Grenzbote
Pressburg, September 2, 1939

Saturday morning a Jewish attack occurred on Hunter's Lane against two FS men, during which both, the twenty-four-year-old Josef Zimmerman and the twenty-year-old student Julius Fo-letar, suffered injuries and had to be removed to the hospital by ambulance.

*Provided in the original German and translated into English by Ernest E. Kovary, who was chief of the translation section in the U.S. Mission to Berlin, Germany, in 1946–47.

Concerning this incredible incident, which proves again how indolently and provocatively Jewry dares to behave here, we received the following details.

THE COURSE OF THE ATTACK

About 10:00 a.m., the FS man Josef Zimmerman was passing unsuspecting through Hunter's Lane, while Julius Foletar, who is also an FS man, happened to come through the street a few houses behind. Suddenly, he noticed that two Jews jumped from house #22, grabbed Zimmerman from behind, and, beating him, dragged him into the lobby. Foletar immediately ran to the aid of his comrade, who was already lying on the ground while the two Jews, their faces distorted in a rage, were blindly hitting him while he was desperately defending himself. Foletar threw himself upon the Jewish gangsters, who, surprised, let go of their helpless victim, who, dazed from the attack and groaning from pain, was stumbling out the door. The next instant the Jews threw themselves with joint forces on Foletar, whom they also injured badly. Foletar had just as little chance as Zimmerman to defend himself properly against the two of them. Furthermore, hearing the noise, a third Jew rushed to the scene, armed with a ski, and also assaulted Foletar, who was lying on the ground.

Hearing the commotion, a passerby rushed in who took the injured Zimmerman into his care, freed Foletar, and in justified anger thrashed the Jews and handed them over to the police. They were identified as the master furrier Olivio Kovary and his two sons, Ernest and Tibor, who attempted to lie during questioning by the police—but they were proven guilty upon the testimony of many witnesses. After they were booked, all three Jews were placed under arrest and taken to the court-prison. Both victims of the attack were taken by ambulance to the state hospital, where Zimmerman was diagnosed as having a broken arm and a series of other injuries and in the case of Foletar severe cuts and lacerations of the head, face, and other parts of his body.

SUBVERSIVE ACTIVITIES OF THE JEWS

This incredible incident furnished clear and convincing proof that it is again and again the Jews who provoke unrest and in this manner work hand in glove with the enemies of the state toward its destruction. In these difficult hours of historical world events, when Germans and Slovaks are marching shoulder to shoulder in exemplary discipline for their just cause, it is precisely the Jews who are spreading the most mindless atrocity stories in their cunning manner—as is reported to us repeatedly.

Ernest Kovary picks up the story: "The Slovak police sat my father down. They asked him his date and city of birth. He responded, 'Baltimore, United States of America.' They did not know what to do with him. So they called the federal prison and sent us there. Dr. Kotska, the head of the Slovak federal prisons, came to meet and interview us personally. We knew if they would have freed us the Slovaks would have lynched us. You see, the Germans influenced people this way. We were all locked up separately. In the middle of the night, a police car came and took us to the federal prison. My brother declined to eat the meal they provided for us because it was not kosher. Eventually, they gave us kosher food. We were incarcerated for several days.

"After ten days, we were placed in the same cell. My father was a former soldier in the Austro-Hungarian army, and with time on his hands in the cell, he made his bunk in true military fashion. He even made lines in the top cover with a toothbrush. This impressed the guards. Many other guards came to look. We developed a good reputation in the prison. Slovak law mandated that within three weeks we had to be charged or released after signing a paper stating that we would appear at trial. Again, in the middle of the night we were taken out of the cell, given our clothing and personal possessions, and told to sign a paper that we would reappear for trial. The prison secretary winked and said, 'All you need is a good visa.' We were taken out of a side door, not the front door, because the Germans were watching. My mother was waiting for us there with a car.

"My father, brother, and I went to the countryside, to my grandmother's house in Trnava, and then to Nitra. My mother stayed in Bratislava; she was not in trouble. In the beginning of December, we received a coded telegram that the Slovak police were looking for us. It meant one thing: we had to escape. My uncle hired a Hungarian farmer who knew the border. On the night of December 12, 1939, we made our escape. The ground was not yet frozen, so we had to tromp through muddy fields across the border. A cab met us in a prearranged location, Nove Zamky [in an area of Slovakia that at the the time was occupied by Hungary]. We had a distant relative living there. We found their home and knocked on the door. My cousin asked, 'Who is there?' We answered that we were relatives of my grandmother Maria [who later died with other family members in Auschwitz]. They took us in and we stayed for a time.

"My father went to Budapest and acquired a ten-day pass to stay. He went to the office for foreigners and the bureaucrat in charge told him not to extend the pass; those who extended were tossed out onto the border. In the meantime, my mother had notified the American consulate. They could not locate my father's file, but had a 1936 letter from the same consulate that indicated that my father had registered as a United States citizen along with his family. Unfortunately, the visa was first sent to Prague, but we were extremely lucky to then have it forwarded to Budapest. We took a train on Saturday, breaking the Sabbath, to meet my mother. Our rabbi approved the journey, stating that it was a life-and-death matter.

"My mother was escorted to the border by the same Hungarian farmer who had escorted us several weeks before, but they were both arrested by the military. She had American dollars sewn into her coat, which was a crime against the state, so she burned them as she was being escorted by the military. The military sent for a woman to body-search her. While she was waiting to be searched, she was sitting next to a wood-burning stove and had the opportunity to burn the money. My mother knew our lives depended on these visas. When questioned by an anti-Semitic military official, she said she had visas for her family. She upbraided the officer, asking him in front of everyone, what did he have against Jews? She shamed him into letting her go. She bribed a border guard with her remaining money, then she found a Jewish woman with an agency who helped reunite her with us.

"Eventually we all made it to Genoa, Italy, and from there we sailed to the United States on the *Conte di Savoy*, the next-to-last ship to leave Italy prior to Italy's entering the war. We arrived on February 29, 1940, in New York Harbor. I joined the U.S. army on October 3, 1941, without formally being a U.S. citizen. I went through basic training at Fort Knox, and although they wanted to send me to Africa because I spoke French, I told them I also spoke German, and they reserved me for Europe. I served as a translator throughout the war.

"After the war, I continued to work within the occupation zone. One day in 1946, I decided to visit Dr. Kotska, who had us released from the Slovak prison. I learned that he had hidden two Jews in his villa during the war. I visited him in the prison, which he had resumed working in. I was dressed in uniform, and when I asked him, 'Do you remember me?' he looked at me without recognizing me. When I announced my name, Kovary, he recognized me immediately. Would you believe he became attorney general of Czechoslovakia? After the war I knew Imi moved to Israel, but I was not sure how to get in touch with him. I wish I had."

Ernest resides in Queens, New York. He worked as a United Nations translator after the war. Ernest remains a pillar of his community and a model of good citizenship—a true *kravist*.

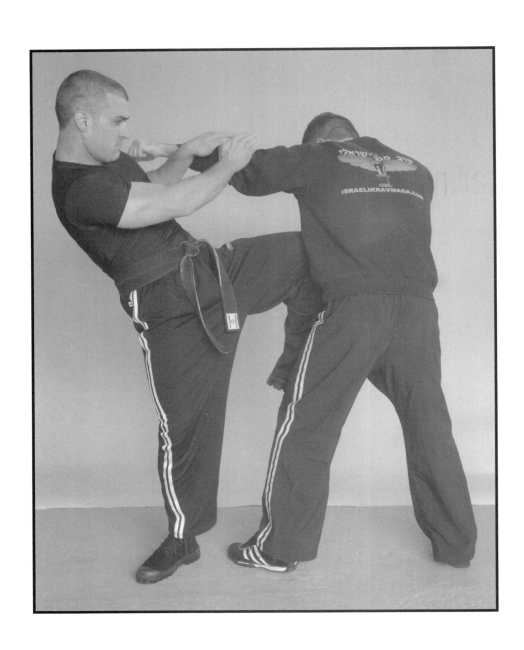

CHAPTER 3

Mastering Upper-Body Strikes and Defenses

Any combative strike will have more force if you accelerate your speed in combination with a total body-weight shift as you extend your personal weapons through your target. The best way to practice these combatives—as with all techniques—is in stages. Each stage must be isolated, practiced, and perfected. As you master the stages, you can combine them for the whole technique. Using a mirror will help you monitor your form. Each move will be explained in detail and illustrated so that you will know how to maneuver. It is difficult to portray the moves in two dimensions, but remember that any combative strike requires all the parts of your body to move in concert.

Many parts of your body, including your hands, forearms, elbows, knees, shins, and head, can be used as personal weapons. There is a distinct advantage in using the hard parts of your body, such as your elbows, knees, and feet, as weapons against your attacker's vulnerable body parts.

Attacking an opponent's soft vital tissues, especially the eyes, throat, and groin, is one of the surest ways to end the fight, and these targets are emphasized in *krav maga*. You know your body's sensitive spots. If you lightly touch yourself in the eye without closing the lid, you will immediately feel your eyeball tense and begin to water. If you have inadvertently hit yourself in the groin or landed on a bicycle bar the wrong way, you know the result. Lightly tap yourself in the throat and you will feel the sensitivity immediately.

Remember, striking someone in the throat can have serious and perhaps fatal consequences. Of course, this is why we are so adamant about protecting our own throats, along with our other vital body parts. The following strikes must only be used if you fear for life or limb.

These strikes are commonly employed from an intermediate range. As with other upper-body strikes, hip and weight movement are essential to take advantage of your body's core strength and mass and deliver reach and power. The striking hand or forearm must also be properly positioned and aligned.

No matter what type of upper-body strike you deliver, shifting your body weight forward to deliver your strike will allow you to place all of your body weight behind the strike, connecting with greater force. Here are some tips for striking effectively.

- **Use your entire body.** As you strike, move the entire body in concert, using your entire torso. As you propel all of your strength and body weight through the strike, you'll maximize your strike's impact.
- **Breathe.** Exhale as you deliver the strike. Some people like to use a bloodcurdling cry as they strike. Either technique—the cry or the exhale—will prepare your body for both delivering a strike and receiving a strike. Exhaling facilitates oxygen transfer to your muscles, tempers your movements to keep you in control, and creates a vacuum in your lungs to defend against a counterstrike to your midsection.
- **Aim for vulnerable targets.** You'll get more for your effort if you strike at the vulnerable targets discussed above.

Straight Front and Rear Punches Reviewed

This strike is a core upper-body combative targeting the nose, jaw, or throat.

Stand in the left outlet stance with your hands in loose fists (see the chapter opener photo). Step forward with your left foot and pivot your rear heel outward. Do not jump at the same time with both feet, as you will lose stability. There is a brief pause between the steps as your entire body launches forward, driving your hip through the punch. Simultaneously extend your left arm, jabbing your fist toward your target. As your arm extends to deliver the punch, tighten your fist. Make contact with your palm parallel to the ground. Raise your left shoulder and tuck your chin to protect your jaw and neck. After striking, return to the left outlet stance. Practice at first by using an open hand and simulating the motion of pushing someone. Then close your fist and duplicate the motion. The idea, as with all combatives, is to refine your body's natural motion.

For the rear punch, stand in the left outlet stance with your hands in loose fists. Pivot your right leg slightly on the ball of the foot as you drive your hips, right (rear) shoulder, and right arm forward toward your target. Tuck your chin into your right shoulder to protect it from an incoming strike. Again, simulate pushing someone with an open hand and then perform the motion again by closing your fist. To practice the combination, let both hands dangle loose as you extend your arms in a natural motion with proper hip pivoting. After you feel comfortable with this loose wrist and hand posture, make a fist and execute proper punches.

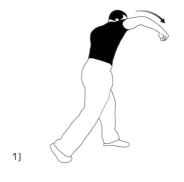
1)

The Over-the-Top Punch

The over-the-top punch attacks your opponent from a slightly vertical angle, slamming down on your opponent's eye socket, nose, or jaw.

Your body movement is similar to an over-the-top elbow, where your striking arm moves high to low and slams down on your target. This strike is especially effective when you are able to trap an opponent's forward arm with your forward arm to bring down his defense while simultaneously delivering the strike to his exposed head.

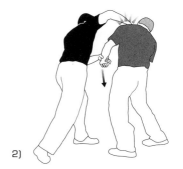
2)

Front Straight Web Strike to the Throat

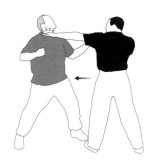

When using this direct and fast strike, aim for the throat and more specifically the windpipe. If your timing and accuracy are correct, this can be a devastating first-strike option.

The web strike uses the webbing of your hand between your forefinger and thumb to strike an opponent's throat and windpipe. By keeping the hand parallel to the ground, you create a thin striking tool capable of getting under an opponent's chin. Stand in the left outlet stance with your hands in loose fists. Similar to the initial movement in straight punches, step forward with your left foot and quickly draw your rear heel slightly in and back. You are not jumping at the same time with both feet. There is a brief pause between the steps as your entire body launches forward. Extend your left arm, thrusting the web of your hand through the target. Make contact with your palm parallel to the ground. Raise your left shoulder and tuck your chin to protect your jaw and neck. Keep your other hand up, protecting yourself, and be prepared to launch another combative move. After striking, return to your left outlet stance.

You must be accurate and extremely careful with this strike because if you do not hit with the web and bone just below your index finger, you may break your thumb. Using your fingers or the web of your hand to strike requires practice. One way to practice this strike is to strike your own thigh just above the kneecap to ensure you know how to properly position the hand.

Rear Straight Web Strike to the Throat

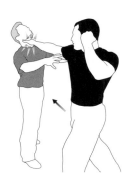

When using this direct and fast strike, aim for the throat and more specifically the windpipe.

Stand in the left outlet stance with your hands in loose fists. Pivot your right leg slightly on the ball of the foot as though you are pushing through a wall. Drive your hips, right (rear) shoulder, and web of your right hand forward and through your target. Tuck your chin into your right shoulder to protect it from an incoming strike. Keep your left hand up, protecting yourself, and be prepared to launch another combative move.

COMBINATION PUNCH AND WEB STRIKE DRILL

A combination drill will allow you to practice the web strike technique along with straight punches to complement both striking options. The straight punches jolt the opponent's head back to expose the throat for the web strike. The drill can be performed with a smaller target pad held by a partner. Your partner should hold the hand pad straight to face you and then, after absorbing your straight punch, instantly turn the pad to the side, exposing the side of the pad for a narrower striking surface that simulates the throat so you can practice your web strike.

1. From the left outlet stance: 20 left straight punches and 20 right rear straight web strikes. Repeat the drill from the right outlet stance 20 times.
2. From both the left and right outlet stances: Create and vary combinations as you feel comfortable. Thinking through different combinations will help you master the techniques and build the base for *retzev*.

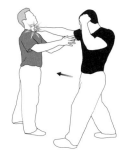

Knuckle Edge Strike to the Throat

When using this direct and fast strike, aim for the throat and more specifically the windpipe. This strike is usually set up by a previous combative.

This combative is similar to the web strike to the throat, except you are using curled fingers and the knuckles as you would use them to knock on a door. The upper- and lower-body movements are the same as the straight punch and web strike except that the striking area of your hand changes. As with the web strike to the throat, you must be careful to align your hand properly. This move will have a devastating effect on the opponent's throat.

COMBINATION PUNCH AND KNUCKLE EDGE STRIKE

This drill combines straight punches and knuckle strikes to the throat, similar to the previous straight punch and web strike combination drill. As with the straight punch and web strike combination, the straight punch jolts the opponent's head back to expose the throat for the knuckle edge strike. The drill can be performed with a hand pad held by a partner. The partner should hold the hand pad straight to face you for both strikes. Be careful with the knuckle edge strike because this strike is designed to target soft tissue and some target pads can be unforgiving.

1. From the left outlet stance: 20 left straight punches and 20 right knuckle edge strikes. Repeat the drill from the right outlet stance 20 times.
2. From both the left and right outlet stances: Create and vary combinations as you feel comfortable. Thinking through different combinations will help you master the techniques and build your *retzev* base.

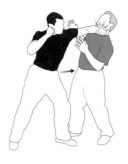

Straight Front Forearm Strike

When using this short, direct, and rapid strike, aim for the throat, jaw, or nose. With your body weight behind it and with proper footwork, this technique is extremely powerful for knocking your opponent back, especially if you strike the throat.

Stand in the left outlet stance with your hands in loose fists. Step forward with your left foot while lifting your left arm parallel to your chest, exposing the outer edge of your forearm. The upper- and lower-body movements are similar to the right rear straight punch, web strike, and knuckle edge strike except for, of course, the striking area. As your outer forearm extends to deliver the strike, tighten your fist, stepping forward to launch your full body weight through the strike. Make sure to step with both feet and thrust off the ball of the rear foot. Raise your left shoulder and tuck your chin to protect your jaw and neck. Keep your other hand up, protecting yourself, and be prepared to launch another combative. After striking to the throat, jaw, or nose, return to your left outlet stance.

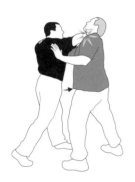

Straight Rear Forearm Strike

This combative is the forearm strike targeting the nose, jaw, or throat but done with the rear (right) arm.

Stand in the left outlet stance with your hands in loose fists. Pivot your right leg slightly on the ball of the foot as you drive your hips, right (rear) shoulder, and outer forearm (dropping perpendicular) toward your target. Tuck your chin into your right shoulder to protect it from an incoming attack. Keep your left hand up, protecting yourself, and prepare to launch another combative. The lower-body pivot and weight shift is the same as the rear straight punch, web strike, and knuckle strike.

COMBINATION FOREARM STRIKE DRILL

A combination drill will allow you to practice the technique. This combination is highly effective in knocking an opponent backward. Using a heavy bag to develop power, a sparring partner for accuracy, or a mirror for overall technique review, practice the following combinations:

1. From the left outlet stance: In alternation, 20 left forearm and 20 right rear forearm strikes. Repeat the drill from the right outlet stance.
2. From the left outlet stance: 20 left forearm and 20 right rear web strikes (or knuckle edge) strikes. Repeat the drill from the right outlet stance.
3. From both the left and right outlet stances: Create and vary combinations as you feel comfortable. Thinking through different front and rear combinations will help you master the techniques and build the base for *retzev*.

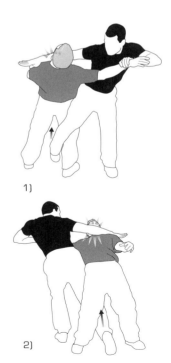

1)

2)

Clothesline Strike to the Throat

This attack thrusts the forearm into the opponent's throat.

You will strike your opponent in his throat by stepping forward and to his side. *Keep your elbow slightly bent.* If you do not, you will injure yourself by hyperextending your elbow. Contact is made with the inner forearm (thumb side) thrusting forward.

You may practice this drill with a heavy bag or a partner holding a hand pad or kicking pad. Make sure your partner holds the pad out and away from the face to avoid receiving an inadvertent strike to the face with the bone just below the pointer finger, known as a ridge-hand strike.

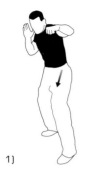

1]

Front Half-Roundhouse Punch

When using this powerful, slightly off-angle strike, aim for the nose, jaw, or throat.

The half-roundhouse punch attacks your opponent with tremendous force. This punch differs from the straight punch because the arm does not shoot out directly toward the target or face-to-face, but rather comes from a slight angle or off angle. To facilitate the off-angle strike punch, the punching side of your body will pivot into the strike while your non-punching shoulder will angle slightly away. This pivoting motion incorporates your deltoid muscles into the strike.

Stand in the left outlet stance with your hands in loose fists. Step forward with your left foot and quickly draw your rear heel slightly outward. You are not jumping at the same time with both feet. There is an ever-so-brief pause between the steps as your entire body launches forward. Simultaneously extend your left arm forward with the elbow coming up and slightly away from your body, thrusting your fist and left hip toward your target. As your arm extends to deliver the punch, tighten your fist. Make contact with the first two knuckles of your hand, keeping it parallel to the ground. Raise your left shoulder and tuck your chin to protect your jaw and neck. After striking, return to your left outlet stance. Keep your other hand up, protecting yourself, and be prepared to launch another combative. For this strike, be sure to keep your wrist properly aligned and strong.

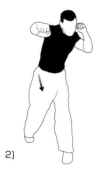

2]

Rear Half-Roundhouse Punch

Similar to the front half-roundhouse punch, this technique best targets the nose, jaw, or throat.

From the left outlet stance, this movement is similar to the front half-roundhouse punch, but your body is pivoting to the left as you attack with the rear arm. Pivot your right leg slightly on the ball of the foot while simultaneously extending your right arm forward with the elbow coming up and slightly away from your body, thrusting your fist toward your target. As you drive your hips, right (rear) shoulder, and arm forward and through your target, tighten your fist. Make contact with the first two knuckles of your hand, keeping it parallel to the ground. Keep your other hand up, protecting yourself, and be prepared to launch another combative. Tuck your chin into your right shoulder to protect it from an incoming strike.

COMBINATION PUNCH DRILL

A combination drill will allow you to practice the half-roundhouse technique along with straight punches. This drill can also combine straight punches, half-roundhouse punches, roundhouse punches, and uppercuts. These combinations are highly effective and are a good foundation to begin *retzev* upper-body combatives. Using a heavy bag to develop power, a sparring partner for accuracy, or a mirror for overall technique review, practice the following combinations:

1. From the left outlet stance: 20 front half-roundhouse and 20 rear half-roundhouse punches. Repeat the drill from the right outlet stance.
2. Combinations from the left outlet stance: 20 front/rear straight punch and front/rear half-roundhouse combinations (two straight punches followed by two half-roundhouse punches is one combination). From the right outlet stance: 20 front/rear straight punch and front/rear half-roundhouse combinations (two straight punches followed by two half-roundhouse punches is one combination).

Continued

3. Combinations from the left outlet stance: 20 front straight punches; 20 rear half-roundhouse punches and front roundhouse combination punches. From the right outlet stance: 20 front straight punches; 20 rear half-roundhouse punches and 20 front roundhouse punches.

4. Combinations from the left outlet stance: 15 front/rear straight punch, front/rear half-roundhouse punch, and front/rear roundhouse punch combinations (two straight punches followed by two half-roundhouse punches followed by a front/rear roundhouse is one combination). Repeat from the right outlet stance, beginning with the right arm.

5. From the left outlet stance: 10 front/rear straight punch, front/rear half-roundhouse punch, front/rear roundhouse punch, front/rear uppercut combinations (two front/rear straight punches followed by two front/rear half-roundhouse punches followed by two front/rear roundhouses followed by two left/right uppercuts is one combination). Repeat from the right outlet stance.

6. From both the left and right outlet stances: Create and vary combinations as you feel comfortable. Thinking through different combinations will help you master the techniques and build your *retzev* base.

Chops

The chop is used on whatever opening your opponent gives you. Targets usually include the kidneys, throat, neck, and nose. Contact is made with the fleshy part of your hand just above where the hand joins the wrist on the pinky side of your hand in a choplike motion. This can stun and injure your opponent. There are two basic types of chops: inward and outward. You may also use the forearm to attack the neck should the distance be too short to execute a chop.

Inward Chop

This technique best targets the sides of the neck (carotid arteries), kidneys, neck, and nose.

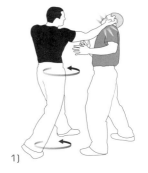

To deliver an inward chop strike with your rear arm, keep your elbow close to your side and bent at approximately 45 degrees. Begin in your left outlet stance with your hands protecting your face. As you deliver the rear chop, pivot on the balls of both feet in the same direction as the chop. This will increase the power of the strike as your lower body and hips move in tandem with your torso and shoulders to generate power. Your wrist will fold back so that the lower "knife" edge, the fleshy underside of the palm and bone just above the wrist joint, makes contact. The positioning resembles the knuckle edge strike to the throat except the wrist is slightly turned out. Keep your other hand up, protecting yourself, and be prepared to launch another combative. The correct way to chop is to keep your forearm and hand semi-tense just prior to impact, when you will then strengthen the entire arm and hand together.

The Outward Chop

This technique best targets the sides of the neck (carotid arteries), throat, and nose.

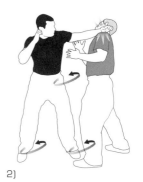

The outward chop uses the same striking surface as the inward chop; however, the wrist is not bent and the hand and forearm are in alignment. As you deliver the chop, you will pivot the front foot in the same direction as the chop so that your toes turn past the target. As you pivot on the ball of your foot, turn the rest of your body, but keep your eyes on the target. Adjust your rear foot slightly to accommodate your front foot's movement. Keep your rear hand up in a fighting position. As in the inward chop, keep the forearm and hand semi-tense until the arm and hand are fully strengthened at the moment before impact. The outward chop is also useful because it keeps a brace between you and your opponent to prevent him from slipping behind you for a takedown or throw.

The following summarizes your chop options and movements. From your regular left outlet stance the following body movements for the chop will apply. Remember that the feet always pivot in the same direction.

1. Inward chop with front (left) arm palm up: Pivot inward on the ball of the front foot, with the rear leg moving in the same direction of the chop—to the right—to accommodate the movement. The rear leg will also pivot slightly outward in the direction of the chop, moving on the ball of the foot.

2. Inward chop with rear (right) arm palm up: Pivot outward on the ball of the front foot while pivoting inward on the ball of the foot of the rear leg in the same direction as the chop.

3. Outward chop with front (left) arm palm down: The same movement as #2 except you are striking with the front arm, holding it parallel to the ground.

4. Outward chop with rear (right) arm palm down: The same movement as #3 but you are striking with the rear arm outward, holding it parallel to the ground.

5. Double chop: Using a front chop palm down followed immediately by a rear chop palm up to the same target. The double chop requires good timing, as the outside chop is delivered with the inside chop immediately following it.

COMBINATION DOUBLE CHOP STRIKE DRILL

This double chop combination is highly effective in debilitating an opponent. Using a heavy bag to develop power, a sparring partner for accuracy, or a mirror for overall technique review, practice the following combinations:

1. From the left outlet stance: 20 left outward and right inward double chop strike combinations. Repeat the drill from the right outlet stance, beginning with the right arm.
2. From both the left and right outlet stances: Create and vary combinations, incorporating chops as you feel comfortable. Thinking through different combinations will help you master the techniques and build the base for *retzev*.

Whipping Blows

This technique principally targets one of the opponent's eyes, while the throat can serve as a secondary target.

Contact with your opponent's eye is made with the pointer and middle finger together, keeping your other fingers loose. Loosen your whipping hand's wrist and let your hand snap at the target eye as though you were whipping someone in the eyes with a towel (an effective technique in its own right). The whip is an easy technique to perform; however, your fingers are vulnerable to injury if your distance or target is inappropriate. Nevertheless, the strike can be used with great effect, especially to distract or stun an opponent and as a setup for additional strikes or to make your escape while the attacker is temporarily blinded.

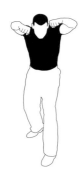

Anti-Group Elbow

This technique targets the jaw, throat, nose, or any other part of the face.

The anti-group elbow is employed when you must make your escape from multiple assailants. You must look for a seam or opening between two opponents in a group confrontation and exploit the seam to make your escape. In *krav maga*, try never to put yourself between two assailants. If you must, place yourself in this vulnerable position for only a split second as you make your escape. *Remember, you must always maneuver to the dead side,* where you are behind the opponent's near shoulder or facing his back. The positioning of your arms is similar to two simultaneous half-roundhouse punches, except one fist (generally the left when beginning from the left outlet stance) is higher than the other. Your striking points on your arms are your fists and elbows. This is so that if you make contact with both arms against opponents flanking you, your fists do not collide. You must tuck your chin and bull your neck by raising your shoulders to protect against blows to the head. Your head, if necessary, can also serve as a modified battering ram. Once you are properly positioned, run and burst through your opponents to safety.

This technique can be practiced with two partners holding two kicking pads high and away from their bodies. Hand pads may also be used; however, kicking pads provide a larger target and additional safety factor for your partners holding the pads.

Inside Defenses Against Straight Punches

Krav maga combines, whenever possible, a deflection with a body defense to avoid an attack (including those with a weapon) and uses *retzev* counterattacks to neutralize the threat. The hand should always lead the body; thus the arm deflection should precede by a fraction of a second the body's defensive movement. This movement "off the line" provides a double layer of protection: redirecting a threat while at the same moment moving yourself away from the threat.

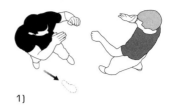

1)

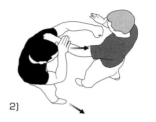

2)

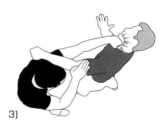

3)

Inside Sliding Parry Against a Straight Front Punch While Stepping Off the Line

This defense allows you to deflect an incoming punch from either side while simultaneously moving away from the punch and delivering your own straight punch counterattack to the throat, chin, or nose.

From your left outlet stance, step to your right with your right foot while bringing your cupped right hand diagonally across your face close to your left shoulder. This hand will again lead the body defense, redirecting the opponent's punch by sliding down your opponent's left arm while your left arm delivers a half-roundhouse counterpunch to your opponent's throat, chin, or nose. You will achieve dead-side positioning. The key is to deflect and step off the line moving both feet together. Do not lunge; keep your feet together and the same distance to the opponent. This defense is readily followed up by trapping the opponent's left arm and delivering a left straight knee to the groin or midsection followed by a right over-the-top elbow (similar in movement to the over-the-top punch but instead using the elbow) to the back of the neck. Additional *retzev* combatives should follow.

Note: You may also step to the left by leading with your left leg. In essence, you are sliding with your left foot rather than stepping with your right. However, you will not achieve the preferred dead-side positioning.

Inside Sliding Parry Against a Straight Rear Punch While Stepping Off the Line

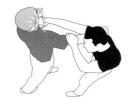

1) Top side, reverse view

This defense allows you to deflect an incoming punch from either side while simultaneously moving away from the punch and delivering your own straight punch counterattack to the throat, chin, nose, midsection, or groin.

From your left outlet stance, step to your left while bringing your cupped left hand diagonally across your face close to your right shoulder. Your hand will lead your body defense, redirecting your opponent's punch by sliding down your opponent's right arm while your right arm delivers a half-roundhouse counterpunch to the throat, chin, or nose. The key is to deflect and step off the line, moving both feet together. Do not lunge; keep your feet moving forward together. You may also punch low to the attacker's body, targeting his liver or delivering a hand strike to his groin. (These last two counterstrikes are useful against attackers who have a height advantage and you cannot readily reach their head to counterattack.) This defense is readily followed up by trapping the opponent's right arm and delivering a right straight knee to the groin or midsection followed by a left over-the-top elbow to the back of the neck. Additional *retzev* combatives should follow, including multiple takedown options to land an opponent hard on his head.

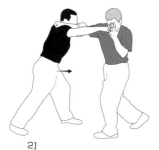

2)

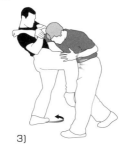

3)

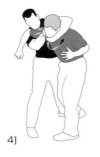

4)

Note: The illustration shows retzev follow-through involving a collar choke. Chokes will be covered in chapter 6. This particular choke involves a half nelson and hold while simultaneously securing the shirt and reaching around with the other arm to secure the shirt choke. Another choke option from this technique is a standing triangle choke (not depicted). Slip your counterpunch arm around the attacker's neck, placing your bicep against one of the main arteries carrying blood to the brain (the right and left carotids) while trapping the attacker's shoulder against the artery on the other side and clamping down in a figure four to execute a

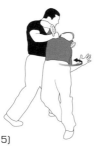

5)

blood choke, as found in chapter 6. Lastly, a number of strong takedowns are available from this triangular choke position, including taking the attacker down into formidable choke positions on the ground.

For both inside sliding parry defenses, if you misread the assailant's straight punch—for example, he throws a right instead of a left—stepping off the line properly will still allow the defense to work. You will have avoided the punch with a body defense (stepping off the line of attack) while counterattacking. In essence, you will "split" the attacker's hands with your counterpunch. The immediate danger is that you are still presenting your live side to your opponent, or he still may have the ability to mount an effective counterattack. The preferred defense is always to move to his dead side, minimizing his ability to counterattack.

The inside sliding parry defenses can be used when on the ground and an attacker is between your legs (a position widely known as the guard). The key is a strong body defense, either moving away or with your dead side to the punch, with a proper slide and simultaneous counterpunch. A closed guard will also help you with a body defense as you shift your hips to unbalance the assailant with your pincered legs as he launches his punches. Be sure to slide fully up the arm as you simultaneously counterpunch to set up additional combatives including, but not limited to, a short hook to the head or throat, or positioning yourself on your side for a straight arm bar (as covered in chapter 6), or a shoulder lock with your legs.

Inside L Block Against a Straight Rear Punch While Stepping Off the Line

This defense, similar to the inside sliding parry, allows you to deflect an incoming straight right punch from either side while simultaneously moving away from the punch, trapping your opponent's arm, and delivering your own straight punch counterattack to the throat, chin, or nose.

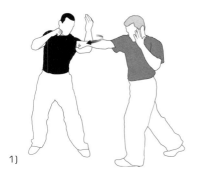
1)

From your regular left outlet stance, your front (left) deflection arm, bent at approximately an 80-degree angle, will lead the body to parry the opponent's right straight punch while making a subtle sidestep. The parrying movement covers no more than six inches and will lead the body defensive movement. This is not an uncontrolled swipe or grab at the attacker's incoming arm (a common mistake when first learning the technique). The defensive arm uses the arm from pinky to elbow to deflect any change in the height of the opponent's strike. The movement rotates the left wrist outward so that your left thumb, kept pressed against the side of the hand with all the fingers pointing up, turns away from you as contact is made with the opponent's arm to redirect the incoming strike. After the parry is made, hook the attacker's arm by cupping your left hand and pinning the arm against the attacker's torso while delivering a counterpunch to the throat or jaw. The goal is to avoid being hit while putting you to the attacker's dead side to continue with *retzev*, be it a takedown and stomp on the head, limb break, or standing combatives.

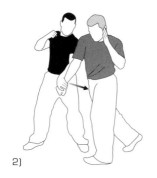
2)

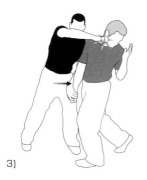
3)

Note: This defense is also used to defend against a straight stab with a weapon.

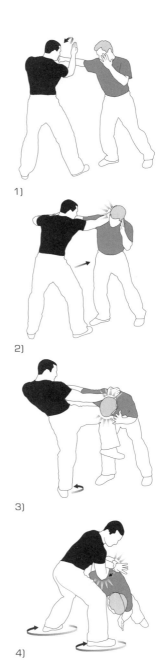

1)

2)

3)

4)

Inside L Block Against a Straight Front Punch While Stepping Off the Line When Opponent Is in an Opposite Stance

This defense, similar to the inside sliding parry, allows you to deflect an incoming straight left punch if you find yourself in a right outlet stance and your opponent is in a left outlet stance. It simultaneously moves you away from the punch and delivers an outside chop to the throat.

From your right outlet stance, bring your right (front) hand, with your arm bent at approximately 80 degrees, to parry the opponent's left straight punch. Again, the parrying movement leads the body defensive movement. It is no more than a six-inch movement diagonally out, not an uncontrolled swipe. After the parry is made, rotate the right arm back and deliver an outside chop (or back fist) to the attacker's neck while securing the opponent's left arm with your left hand. Continue with *retzev*, delivering a right knee to the groin, a right horizontal elbow to the throat, or a right vertical elbow to the back of the neck followed by additional *retzev* combatives.

Note: This L parry may be used against an opponent who is standing to your side if you are both facing the same way. In other words, your attacker tries to attack you from the side, where you might not see him, or to sucker-punch you. You will parry the punch and move to his dead side, unleashing simultaneous retzev combatives.

Outside Defenses Against Straight Sucker Punches

Using an outside block or 360-degree instinctive defense, this technique deflects a straight punch delivered by an opponent standing to your side while you and he are facing in opposite directions.

You will deflect your opponent's incoming straight punch and pivot to his dead side, delivering the following (recommended options):

1. Low body punch, chops, or elbows to kidneys with additional *retzev* combatives
2. Knee to kidneys with additional *retzev* combatives
3. For those who are flexible, a roundhouse kick to the head with additional *retzev* combatives

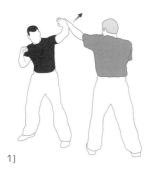

1)

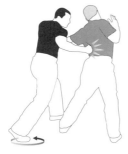

2)

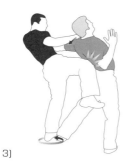

3)

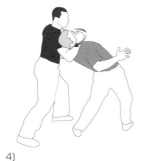

4)

Additional Defenses Against Sucker Punches

An assailant can sucker-punch you, or deliver a straight punch sneak attack, when standing or seated next to you.

This instinctive defense allows you to duck your head into your shoulder while raising your shoulder to protect your head and absorb or deflect the incoming punch. Simply lift your shoulder and tuck your head while leaning away from the punch. A simultaneous side kick to the assailant's knee provides a formidable simultaneous defense and attack option—*krav maga's* fundamental tenet of stopping an attacker. In other words, as you tuck your head and lean back, pick up your near-side leg and deliver a devastating side kick with proper base leg movement by pivoting on the ball of the foot to direct the heel of your base leg toward your opponent for maximum power and reach. This defense works best against an attacker standing to your side but facing in the opposite direction, though it also can be effective against an attacker standing to your side and facing in the same direction. A preferable defense against a sucker punch thrown by an attacker to your side and facing in the same direction is the inside L defense.

> *Note: The inside sliding parry defenses previously introduced may work against this type of attack; however—as with all defenses—timing is crucial. You must step out of the line of attack in time to deflect and counterpunch.*

Inside Defenses Against Left/Right Straight Combinations

Using a sidestep body defense to the left, you will lean away from the incoming left punch (attacker is in a left outlet stance) and simultaneously deliver a rear straight punch followed by a right kick to the groin and *retzev* combatives.

> *Note: This may be done to either side, and you may position your opposite hand in an inside sliding defense for additional protection.*

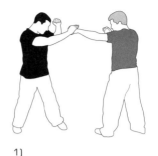

1)

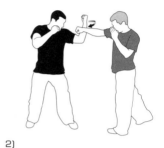

2)

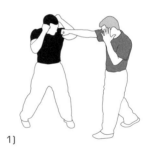

1)

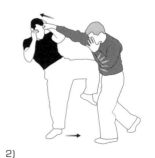

2)

Straight Punch Deflection with Modified L Block and Angled Gunt Option

This defense uses the basic inside punch deflection punch against the knuckle of the opponent's left pinky finger (without a body defense movement), but instead of a second basic deflection with your opposite arm against the opponent's incoming right arm, a forearm or elbow variation deflection with your lead bent arm is useful if you are late defending against the second incoming punch. Immediately after the left modified L block, follow up with a straight counterpunch with your right arm. If the move is executed properly, the elbow deflection can break the attacker's hand. This defense can also be used with a double elbow deflection with both arms.

From your left outlet stance, deflect the opponent's left punch with a parry aiming at the knuckle of his left pinky finger. Then use your right arm, bent at a 90-degree angle, to execute an L block by rotating the arm inward slightly, turning your right palm toward your face, to deflect the punch with the fleshy part of your inner forearm. You have the option of also drawing your right hand into your ear and raising your right elbow to form a defensive shield against the second incoming punch. Counterattack with your own left/right combination, kick, or knee as you see fit, followed by *retzev* combatives. You may also reverse this defense, using an angled gunt against the first strike and a basic deflection against the second strike. Lastly, you may use two gunts with an immediate counterattack using a kick, knee, or immediate upper-body counterattack.

Note: Angled gunts are good for defending against a close, unexpected attack and can defend against an onslaught of different straight, hook, uppercut, and other off-angle punch variations.

Parry Against Straight Punches with Immediate Counterpunch or Roundhouse Kick

This defense uses a parry against the first left punch and intercepts the second punch with a simultaneous parry and immediate countering straight punch.

This explanation assumes both you and your attacker are in left outlet stances. As the left punch comes in, you will parry it with your same-side arm followed by another parry against the second incoming punch with your opposite arm. As soon as you parry the second punch, you will slightly cup your hand to send the second punch's arm away while counterpunching with the same hand that performed the second defense. Follow with knees, elbows, and other *retzev* combatives.

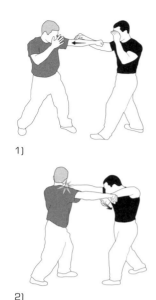

1)

2)

Note: *This defense's block and deflection can be employed to defend against a single straight punch as well, or a same-side deflection and counterpunch using your same arm. You may also deflect a straight punch and deliver a powerful rear roundhouse kick to the attacker's forward leg.*

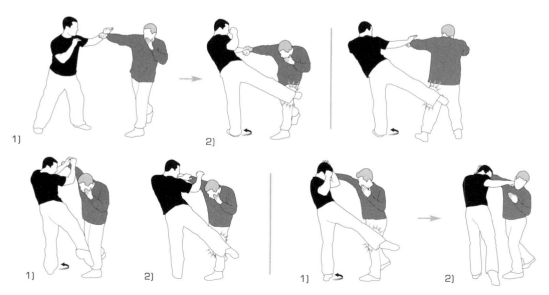

1)   2)   1)

1)   2)   1)   2)

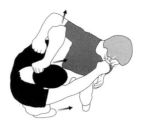

Parallel Gunt Against a Hook Punch

This highly effective defense protects the head from hook punches and high roundhouse kicks to the head.

From the left outlet stance, tuck your chin by burying it into your left shoulder while folding your arm across with your elbow tip pointed out at approximately a 45-degree angle to intercept and block the hook punch at its earliest stage and to act as a shock absorber. Do not fold the arm directly against your head; this avoids an indirect blow to your head through your blocking arm's absorption of the strike. Simultaneously attack the opponent's head or neck with counterstrikes. This placement also sets up a convenient horizontal elbow counterattack, as you can then come across with an elbow strike to the opponent's neck or head. You can also use the elbow tip after the block to draw it parallel to your head and drive forward into the opponent's face. *Keep in mind this defense is not designed for defending against an edged weapon attack.*

STRIKING COMBINATIONS INCLUDING FEINTS

Feints, showing one combative movement but transitioning immediately to another combative, are a decisive tactic to attack your opponent by luring him into the wrong defensive posture or movement.

Striking combinations including feints (partial list)

1. Low straight punches with body defense
2. Low roundhouse/high roundhouse with same-arm and opposite-arm combinations
3. Straight punch and horizontal elbow combination with the same arm
4. Straight punch and horizontal roundhouse combination with the same arm
5. Roundhouse punch with the forward arm and straight punch with the rear arm
6. Feinting roundhouse punch into straight punch
7. Feinting straight punch into roundhouse punch
8. Feinting straight punch into uppercut
9. Any combination of the above

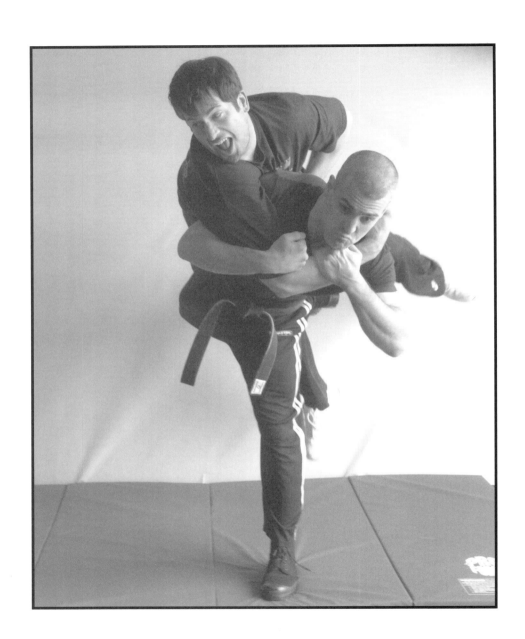

CHAPTER 4

Mastering Lower-Body Strikes and Defenses

Krav maga emphasizes kicks using the ball of the foot, heel, and shin along with knee strikes to the opponent's midsection, groin, and legs. These body parts are highly vulnerable as well as less defensible. A low kick has less chance of being trapped by an opponent than would a high kick, and low kicks are conducive to being interspersed with upper-body combatives.

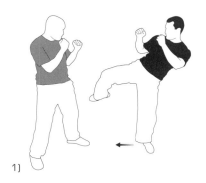
1)

Half-Roundhouse Knee

These powerful combatives attack your opponent's vulnerable thigh using your patella (knee) and shin with your full body weight behind the strike.

Similar to the front and rear knee, your support (base) leg will turn out as you use *glicha* (sliding step) to launch your body weight forward and close the distance to your opponent. Angle your knee and shin at approximately 45 degrees to the ground. As you make contact using your patella and shin, thrust the shin

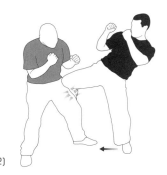
2)

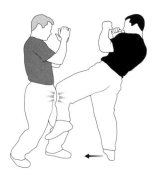

out for added impact and power. You may also add a simultaneous straight punch with your lead arm for a combined upper- and lower-body attack.

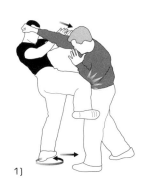

1)

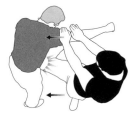

2) Top view

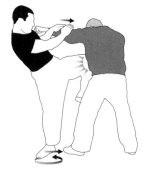

Left punch defense

Two-Handed Sliding Block Against Straight Rear and Front Punches with Knee Attack Stepping Off the Line

This is a devastating counterattack using a two-handed deflection and body defense, with a knee counterattack using your entire body weight into the attacker's groin or midsection.

From your left outlet stance, you will use both arms to deflect the opponent's incoming straight right punch. You will turn both of your arms to your right so that the forearms are facing in the same direction with your hands slightly cupped and palms down. This allows for a strong sliding deflection against the outside of your opponent's right arm. You must again step off the line to your left. As you take the step, you are propelling your knee with your body weight behind it into your opponent's groin or midsection with a modified roundhouse knee. Follow up with an over-the-top elbow slamming down on the back of your opponent's neck, combined with additional *retzev* combatives.

Note: You may also use a variation of this defense if your attacker attempts to sucker-punch you and you are both facing the same direction. Once again, you must step off the line and with a double forearm block deliver a powerful roundhouse knee to his midsection.

Offensive Knee and Trap Against Attacker Standing in Left Outlet Stance

This combined trap and knee combative is designed to catch and control your opponent's arms while delivering a devastating front knee to the opponent's groin, thigh, or midsection followed by additional retzev *combatives.*

If your opponent has his arms close together, trapping him by grabbing and pulling his arms to you can be highly effective. As you grab both of his wrists with your hands, yank him into you as you propel a straight knee into his midsection with a proper 90-degree base (non-kicking) leg turn.

If your opponent has his hands wide apart, you can split his hands by putting your palms together and stabbing your arms between his arms, driving them farther apart as you deliver a straight knee with proper base leg turn.

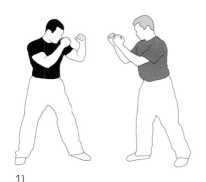

1)

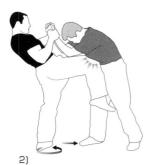

2)

Low Roundhouse Kick Sweep

Sweeps utilize powerful low roundhouse-type kicks to "sweep" an opponent's leg or legs out from under him. The main target is usually the Achilles tendon; however, the knees are also vulnerable to this type of combative.

From your left outlet stance, raise your right (rear) leg and then rotate the knee, thigh, and shin parallel to the ground. Pivot on the ball of your left (base leg) foot while bending the knee slightly so that your body turns to the right, in the direction of

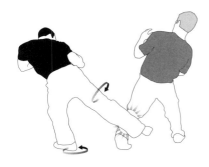

your kneecap. As you bend the knee, your leg will necessarily extend out farther to facilitate sweeping your opponent. Keep your eyes on your target. Continue to pivot and swing around toward your opponent as you straighten and strengthen your kicking leg to kick through your opponent. As with your other combative strikes, your entire weight comes through the kick as your body torques through the target like a hatchet chopping down a tree. When you kick-sweep, your hip must rotate parallel to the ground so that your foot stays parallel to the ground. Lower your center of gravity to target the opponent's Achilles tendon, just above the ankle.

Stepping Side Kick

This extremely powerful combative enables you to cover a longer distance and kick an opponent who is to your side. Targets include the shin, knee, thigh, midsection, or head.

The stepping side kick is an effective combative for striking an opponent at a greater distance using a long step (*secoul*). You "cheat" by positioning your feet almost perpendicular to your opponent, rather than using the left outlet stance, where your feet are positioned at an angle of about 45 degrees to your opponent. Execute the stepping side kick with the front leg, closest to your target. Your rear leg (base leg) crosses behind your front leg as you prepare to launch the kick. Shift your weight to your rear leg, angle your heel toward the opponent, extend your leg parallel to the floor, and make contact with the heel. The stepping leg's heel must face the opponent. While you may lean back slightly because your kicking leg is raised with your thigh parallel to the ground, make sure your weight is coming forward and through your target.

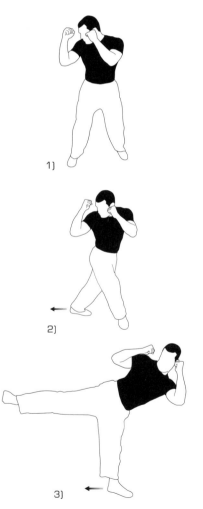

1)

2)

3)

Spinning Sidekick

This tremendously powerful combative enables you to spin and kick an opponent who is to your front or side. This kick is designed to follow your sliding or stepping side kick. This can be a particularly devastating surprise combative targeting the knees, thigh, groin, midsection, or head.

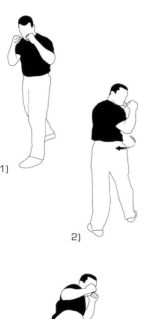

1)

2)

With any spinning offensive strike, your head must turn to see your opponent before you begin the spin. The spin should be very short to allow for a quick turn. The best way to practice—as with all techniques—is in stages. As you master each stage, you can then combine them for the complete technique. Using a mirror will help you monitor your form. For the spinning side kick, face the mirror with your kicking leg to the rear. This differs from the regular sliding and stepping side kicks because in the spinning side kick your rear leg will deliver the kick rather than your front leg. Let's assume you are facing the mirror in your left outlet stance. Step 1 is to turn your left leg so that the side of your foot is parallel to the mirror. Step 2 is to turn your head over your right shoulder as your kicking leg rises. Step 3 is to turn or spin the body and launch the kick. Make sure to perfect the line of the kick to drive your kick straight through your target and not off to the side. This will require practice.

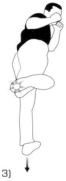

3)

SIDE KICK EXTENSION AND BALANCE DRILL

This drill is designed to enhance your form and balance and also provide a strengthening component. With a partner, stand facing one another in "cheating stances," turning both of your feet perpendicular to your opponent as you would if you were preparing to deliver a side kick. One partner should use his left hand to grab the other partner's left hand, then he should position himself in the initial stage of the kick with his leg cocked and heel resting against the other partner's midsection. Once in position, the partner executing the side kick will extend his leg against the partner, who should moderately resist the push, creating separation between them. Perform the drill on both legs, with each partner taking turns with 10 repetitions per leg.

Defenses Against Straight Kicks

These defenses are designed to counter straight kicks launched against you. Optimally, you will use your front leg to parry the kick, but sometimes a hand defense is necessary. Remember, lowering your hands to defend against a kick can expose you to upper-body strikes, particularly straight punches, so be careful.

Instinctive Inside Deflection with Palm Heel/Forearm Retreat

From a natural stance or open stance facing your opponent, the inside instinctive deflection with palm heel/forearm is designed to redirect a straight kick launched at your groin or midsection while you step back to create distance from the attacker. The defense will work against either a front kick or a rear kick, but it works better against a rear kick (assuming you and your opponent are in left outlet stances) because the defense will bring you to your opponent's dead side. This defense builds on our instinct to swipe away or deflect a threat coming at our body, directing the momentum away from us. Rather than a pure deflection, you will take a step back and position yourself slightly off angle from the incoming kick to deflect it, and then grab the attacker's leg at the Achilles tendon or, if necessary, by the pant leg and pull him into you while executing a powerful rear punch followed by additional retzev *combatives.*

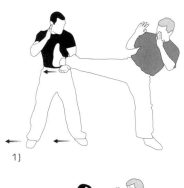

1)

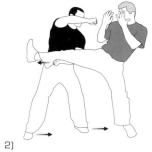

2)

From the left outlet stance, take a rear sidestep to move you off the line while bringing your left arm down with your elbow slightly bent and close to your body to deflect the kick. Keep your hand open with all of the fingers pressed together. The objective is to deflect the attacker's kick slightly above his ankle to move the kick away from you. Any higher and your defense will be too late and it will be extremely difficult to redirect his momentum. When you deflect, try to keep the arm as close as you can to the body to give the arm strength and protect your elbow from being injured. Once the deflection is made, pull your attacker into your counter right straight punch, followed by additional *retzev* combatives.

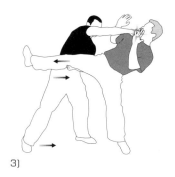

3)

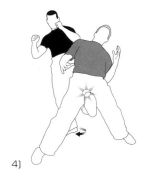

4)

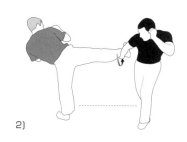

1)

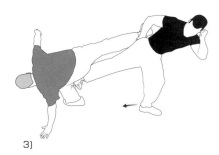

2)

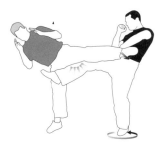

3)

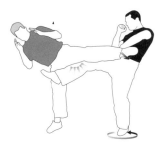

Left kick defense variation

Outside Scoop Defenses Using Hooks

This defense uses a deflection method along with a subtle retreating side-step, using your front arm to deflect incoming kicks to the outside (rather than the inside) while also using a body defense to get off the line. While the rear arm can also be used, it can be dangerous because the incoming kick will be too close to your body at that point to make an effective deflection.

Depending on your opponent's angle, your front arm will either be on the opposite side or the same side as the attacker's kicking leg. Optimally, you would use the opposite-side arm to turn or spin the opponent away from you, allowing you to get to his dead side. If you and your opponent are both in the left outlet stance, you will defend against his rear (right) kick with your right arm and against his front (left) kick with your left arm to turn him away from you and not allow his other leg to have a chance to come at you.

To execute the deflection, bring your arm down and away from your torso using a scoop-type hand alignment with your wrist bent inward and thumb pressed against the hand to deflect the incoming kick slightly above the ankle. If you and your opponent are in the same outlet stance and he kicks with his front leg, as you deflect you can deliver a straight kick with your rear leg.

The danger is that this defense keeps you to your opponent's live side and you must react quickly with a *retzev* counterattack. However, this gives you good defensive flexibility. If you and your opponent are both in the left outlet stance, you will defend against his rear (right) kick with your left arm and his front (left) kick with your left arm.

Note: The instinctive inside defense together with scoop defenses can create effective lead-arm defenses against straight kicks from the rear (inside deflection defense) and straight kicks from the front (outside deflection defense). Remember, your lead arm is closer to the kick, and it can intercept and deflect the kicks sooner.

Inside Deflection Against High Kick

This defense parries a straight high kick to your head. It is similar to the first step of your inside L block against a straight punch (page 49).

From your regular left outlet stance, make a subtle sidestep to your left while bringing your left (lead) hand, with your arm bent at approximately 80 degrees, to parry an opponent's kick to your head using either leg. The parrying movement is no more than a six-inch movement. It is not an uncontrolled swat or grab at the attacker's incoming leg (a common mistake when first learning the technique). The forearm uses a broad deflective surface, from wrist to elbow. The movement rotates the left wrist outward so that your left thumb turns away from you as contact is made with the opponent's leg to redirect the incoming high straight kick. Counter immediately with a *retzev* counterattack.

Sliding Deflection Defense Against Front and Rear Straight Kicks

This venerable defense will take you off the line and allow you to deliver a counterpunch to the attacker's throat, jaw, or nose.

From your regular outlet stance, make a subtle sidestep while punching down across the line of attack to execute a glancing blow and deflect the opponent's incoming kick. Use this diagonal defense regardless of whether it is a front or rear kick. At the

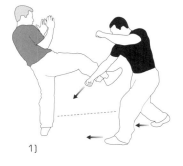

1]

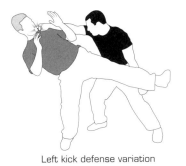

2]

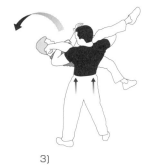

3]

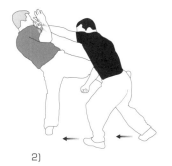

Left kick defense variation

same time deliver a counterpunch to the opponent's throat, jaw, or nose followed by *retzev* combatives. Note that you do not punch the shin. Similar to other *krav maga* deflecting movements, the objective is to redirect the incoming strike away from you while moving off the line. A throw may be incorporated into the defense by hooking the opponent's leg with the crook of your elbow. As you catch the leg, explode up with your knees and hurl the attacker backward. Follow up with additional stomps and *retzev* combatives.

Body Defense and Counterattack Against a Straight Kick by Moving Off the Line

This body defense takes you off the line of attack and uses a counterpunch to stun the attacker.

From the left outlet stance, take a sidestep to your right to avoid a straight kick launched against your midsection while delivering a strong right counterpunch to the opponent's neck, jaw or nose followed by *retzev* combatives. In a sense, you are switching your feet from a left outlet stance to a right outlet stance. This particular technique relies on a body defense. You may also step through (from your left outlet stance) with your right foot, again moving off the line to deliver a right punch to the attacker's head while deflecting with the left.

Defenses Against Side Kicks

Defenses against side kicks are challenging and must reach the kick's height. You must recognize your opponent's positioning as he sets up for a side kick. Remember that when you perform a side kick, you "cheat" in your outlet stance by drawing your front foot perpendicular to your opponent's front leg. Look for this in your opponent's positioning because he may be preparing to do the same to you.

You know from practicing your own side kicks the power and reach this kick can deliver. Keep this in mind when mastering the corresponding defenses.

Stop Kick Against Side Kick

It is possible to deliver a straight stop kick against an opponent's side kick, but it is difficult and your timing must be exceptional. You can deliver a straight kick so that your foot is vertical when intercepting the opponent's kicking foot, which is horizontal.

Outside Scoop Deflection Against Side Kick

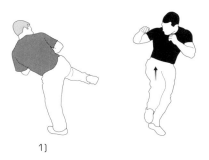

1)

As with the outside scoop deflection you used against the straight kick, you will time the defense to misdirect the opponent's kick while delivering a devastating counterblow to his base leg knee.

You may use the scoop deflection defense as learned against the low straight kick using your forward arm. Rather than scoop at the opponent's ankle, you will scoop at the outside of his heel. This facilitates the defense and allows you to deliver a counter side kick to his knee while reaching his dead side. You will be hard pressed to successfully defend against a side kick from the opposite stance when you are in a left outlet stance and your opponent is in a right outlet stance or vice versa. If your stance does not take you dead side to your opponent, he can readily adjust the kick to defeat the defense. Yet defending against a side kick from an outlet stance where your left (forward) leg is facing the opponent's left (forward) leg is possible. This defense requires you to hook your opponent's incoming heel using your forward arm while raising your forward leg to avoid the incoming low

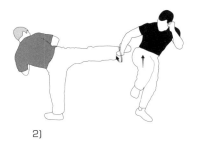

2)

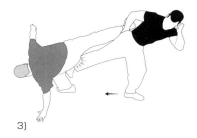

3)

side kick by sweeping aside the opponent's kicking leg by its heel. Your forward arm should turn your palm toward the heel of your opponent's incoming kicking leg. As you sweep aside the kick, you will deliver your own counter side kick to your opponent's base leg. Be sure to sweep your defending arm outside with enough force to deflect a strong incoming side kick.

High Side Kick Defense

To defend against a high side kick to the head, you can use the inside cross parry punch defense to deflect the kick, as you learned to do with a straight kick to the head. Alternatively, you may use a deflection underneath the kick with your forearm while dropping your torso to take your head below the kick (a modified block from a 360-degree instinctive defense where you achieve different blocking positions by moving your arms in a defensive circle) to send it upward, away from your head. This #1 block is similar to the forearm strike except you are angling the strike up to redirect the kick away from your head. An advanced *krav maga* technique employs a sidestep to avoid the kick by using a double forearm block (similar to a horizontal elbow defense) with palms facing in to deflect the kicking leg at the shin.

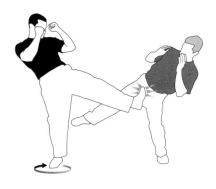

Preemptive Straight Kick Against a Roundhouse Kick

Against any level roundhouse kick, you may peremptorily straight-kick the attacker's groin, followed by additional *retzev* combatives. You may also use a front roundhouse kick to sweep the attacker's base leg with your front leg. It is possible, with good timing, to launch a preemptive straight punch to the opponent's throat, jaw, or nose at the moment your recognize your opponent winding up for the kick. Remember, however, that leg reach is usually longer than arm reach.

Late Leg Defense Against Low Roundhouse Kick

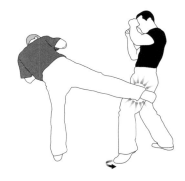

This defense becomes necessary when you do not recognize an incoming low roundhouse kick early enough to defend against it otherwise and must absorb the kick.

If you are late in recognizing the low roundhouse kick to the leg, you can pivot on your front leg, tensing and strengthening the quadriceps muscle to better absorb the kick. This will be painful, but angling your leg (similar to angling your forearm against a high roundhouse kick) will help deflect the kick upward to mitigate its power.

Outside 45-Degree Gunt Defense Against a High Roundhouse Kick

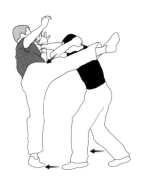

This highly effective defense protects the head from high roundhouse kicks.

Tuck your chin by burying it into your shoulder while bringing your folded arm up to your head with the elbow directed outward at a 45-degree angle (similar to the gunt defense against a hook punch).

Stop Kick Against a Spinning Side Kick

Although it is challenging, with correct timing it is possible to deliver a straight stop kick against an opponent's spinning side kick. You can deliver a straight kick to your opponent's buttocks to stop his spin when he turns his back to initiate the kick. Immediately follow up with *retzev* combatives.

Defenses Against Low Roundhouse Sweeps

Defending against low roundhouse sweeps is important and requires good timing since the trajectory of the sweep is so low. You have a few options:

1. Pick up your front leg
2. Execute a defensive kick (front/back) to the opponent's body
3. Close the distance with hand attacks (requires good timing)
4. Jump or change legs through *tsai-bake* to avoid the sweep

LOWER-BODY DRILLS

Kick/punch combination drills

These are exercises to build the all-important *retzev.*
1. Straight rear kick with step forward (into opposite outlet stance) and punch in one motion
2. Straight front kick forward with step and punch with same-side arm
3. Straight kick to groin from rear and knee to head with same leg
4. Low/high roundhouse combination with same leg
5. Straight kick forward and then knee with other leg
6. Shove opponent backward to unbalance him and deliver low roundhouse sweep
7. Blocking opponent's vision with hand or glove and sweeping
8. Sweeping opponent's base leg when opponent is kicking

Defenses against combinations

1. Defense against straight kick to groin and punch to the face (inside deflections and counterattacks)
2. Defense against roundhouse kick (varying heights) and punches

Kick feint drills

1. Faking roundhouse kick into straight punch (kick does not land)
2. Down-up kicks, when you feint low and kick high
3. Side kick feint into reverse roundhouse
4. Straight kick into high roundhouse kick (kick must be one movement, not two)
5. Side kick by faking a sweep to leg (in one movement, kick almost all the way but pull back slightly to deliver a side kick; must sell commitment to roundhouse kick)
6. Side kick faking front kick (look for opening, high or low)
7. Roundhouse kick into straight kick
8. Regular front or rear kick into side kick
9. Roundhouse feint kick into side kick
10. Straight low kick feint into high roundhouse kick

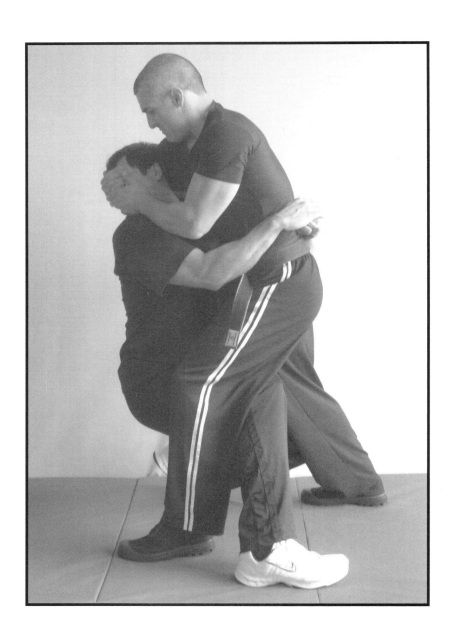

CHAPTER 5

Mastering Releases and Takedown Defenses

Defending against grabs, traps, and takedowns is an indispensable skill. Upper- and lower-body strikes, if improperly executed or if well defended against by your opponent, can place you in a precarious position, resulting in a trap or takedown. Well-executed upper- and lower-body combatives minimize this risk, but there is still a risk, especially if you are fighting against someone who is skilled in ground combat. Keep in mind a few strategies ground-fighting specialists can employ against you:

- An opponent can retreat backward, luring you in, only to lunge low at your legs for a takedown.
- An opponent can close the distance between you by luring you into throwing an upper- or lower-body combative. As you commit to the move, he will change his level and initiate a takedown. *Retzev* allows you to seamlessly combine upper- and lower-body combatives along with evasive action to prevent a takedown.

- An opponent can attack you with upper- and lower-body combatives that may or may not physically connect, but the strategy might be to distract you, setting up an easier takedown.
- Rather than a initiate linear attack, an opponent can "break the angle," crossing up your footwork, or simply position himself to take you down from your dead side.

You must be able to defend against an opponent who is changing his level of attack. Allowing an opponent to successfully change his level provides him with the opportunity to attack your legs with significant force and speed. Successful takedowns often are set up by a combatant using a distraction (usually an upper-body strike feint). While the combative distraction may or may not connect, it will allow the combatant to lower his level with proper posture to protect his head from counterattack. Thus, a strong attack against the legs is made possible, with the combatant keeping his elbows close to his body and gliding forcefully under the opponent's lead arm with his shoulder, making takedown contact at the opponent's hip and thighs.

Release Against Two People Gripping Arms

A quick release against two people gripping your arms involves using either a side kick or a straight kick to counterattack in the knee, groin, or midsection of one attacker and then the other. You can use the same leg for both kicks, or each leg can execute a kick. If a third attacker approaches, you should kick the third attacker first, making sure to turn the hips, which will facilitate your release from the other two assailants.

The Shirt-Hold Pressure and Lock Release

The shirt-hold pressure and lock defense is effective against a one- or two-handed shirt grab. It will rotate the attacker's hand to the inside by applying a joint lock to his shoulder and elbow. Of course, you could simply take down your attacker with combatives, but the goal of this technique is control and compliance.

The shirt-hold pressure and lock release involves moving from a cross grab defense into an arm bar. The same defense is used against a one- or two-handed shirt grab. If the attacker is facing you and grabs with his right hand, you will reach across your chest with your right arm, sliding your hand across your chest to grab the attacker's hand by positioning your palm facing down while trapping the opponent's hand between your hands. By positioning your knuckles down ("thumb to you") with your palm against the back flat side of his hand with your opposite hand also facing down and parallel, you will rotate the attacker's hand down and away. After securing the opponent's hand in this "prayer" hold, rotate your hand down, which will rotate your opponent's hand up. Simultaneously, place downward pressure on the opponent's wrist and forearm using your body weight.

The same basic technique is used for a shirt-hold defense variation in which you use only your arm opposite to the opponent's grabbing arm (if your opponent grabs with his right, you will rotate his arm with your right) to grab and rotate using the same movement as described previously. At the same time, use your same-side (left) hand to pluck out the attacker's arm below the elbow, creating a slight bend in the arm to facilitate downward pressure.

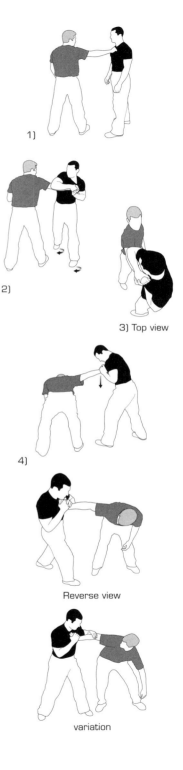

1)

2)

3) Top view

4)

Reverse view

variation

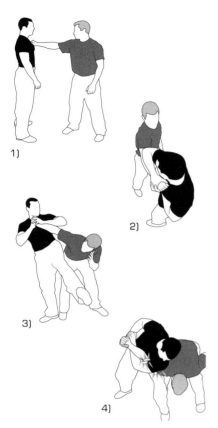

1)

2)

3)

4)

The Shirt-Hold Standing Arm Bar Release

The shirt-hold standing arm bar release against a one- or two-handed shirt hold is a powerful technique that involves applying a joint lock to your attacker's elbow. Once you have applied the lock, dropping your weight down on the elbow joint creates tremendous breaking pressure. Once again, you could simply disengage you attacker with combatives, but the goal here is control.

The shirt-hold standing arm bar involves a cross grab wrist lock or cavalier into a standing arm bar with a step-through to put the opponent facedown. You will cross-grab the attacker's arm, similar to the first shirt-hold release; however, you will step through with the same-side leg to execute a standing arm bar by exerting pressure on the attacker's arm above the elbow while maintaining a strong grip. This also protects you from a groin strike counterattack. You must be close to the attacker's body to maximize the submission hold's effect and minimize possible countermeasures. You may transition to a figure four hold for maximum control.

Defense Against Side Headlock When Attacker Is Forcing the Defender Forward

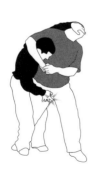

This defense counters an attacker who has put you in a headlock and is driving you forward when you cannot maintain or recover your balance.

Your first option is to lock the attacker's front leg with both your legs, thwarting his ability to drive you forward. Simultaneously, take the arm closest to the attacker's torso and wrap it around the rear of the attacker's shoulder closest to you, embedding a finger in his eye while striking his groin with your other arm.

The second option requires that you set down your outside

knee while bringing your front arm forward to strike the attacker's groin while the other arm grabs the attacker around the hips. You will sit down to roll with the attacker forward and continue your attacks. Following up with a mount to trap his arms to your torso is highly effective along with other *retzev* joint locks and breaks.

Duck Against Choke or Side Headlock

A quick defense against a choke or side headlock is to move underneath, slapping the groin. There is also the option of elbows, chokes, and throws against your attacker.

Release from Blood Choke Variation

If you have turned in toward the crook of the attacker's elbow, continue to turn in toward the attacker's choking arm. Simultaneously, you will sweep the attacker's leg with a rear sweep, forcefully kicking through with the hooked leg (see chapter opening photo).

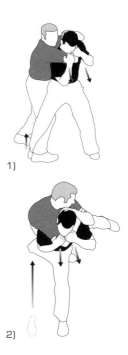

1)

2)

> Note: If the opponent is using a figure four or "professional choke" grip, you must yank down on the crook of the attacker's elbow while clearing the other hand from behind your head.

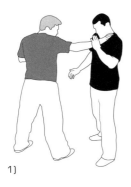

1)

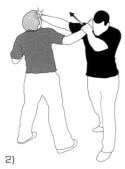

2)

Release from Front Choke While Against a Wall

This choke release is used when you are pressed against the wall and the attacker can exert increased force against you because the wall prevents your evading the choke.

Unlike other front choke release options where you can move backward to aid in removing or plucking the attacker's hands from your throat, here you have no room because of the wall. The attacker can lock his elbows and place tremendous pressure on your throat. If the attacker gets a firm hold on your throat with his thumb(s) on your windpipe, removing his hands with a pluck can cause serious damage. Therefore, you must remove his hand by a cross thrust or push while attacking his eye, followed by additional combatives.

Collar Chokes and Defenses

Collar chokes are highly effective and are defended against in a similar way as with hand chokes to your neck. Tremendous leverage can be created by using your opponent's shirt collar, lapel, or tie against him. While there are ten collar choke variations in the *krav maga* curriculum, we will show one basic collar choke for illustrative purposes.

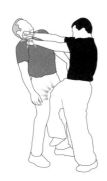

Front and Rear Cross Collar Choke

You are face-to-face with your opponent. For the cross collar choke, place your left hand close to the jugular vein of your opponent. With your right arm grab his clothing close to the other jugular vein. You must acquire a strong grip by punching your knuckles in. Once you have a tight, secure grip, punch across the throat by thrusting your right hand over your left hand.

"Knuckles-in" Collar Choke

For the "knuckles-in" choke, you will insert your hands into your opponent's collar with your thumbs up. While keeping your elbows close and down toward your opponent's shoulders, tighten your grip on the collar and roll your hands in, putting extreme pressure on the carotid arteries to cut off blood flow to the brain.

Defending against collar chokes is similar to defending against chokes with the attacker's bare hands around your neck. Note, however, that these defenses become more difficult because of the strong enabling grip the clothing will allow your opponent. Of course, the best defense is to prevent your opponent from inserting his hands in your collar in the first place.

Front Collar Choke Defenses

These two defenses are similar to krav maga's *other front choke defenses, involving a pluck to release choking pressure coupled with a simultaneous counterattack. Note that due to the nature of the attack you will have to counterattack the opponent's eyes from the outside rather than from between his choking arms.*

Front Collar Choke Defense 1

This defense is used when your legs and knees are not available to counterattack and you still have separation (your attacker is not pressed against you). With your left hand, pluck the attacker's right hand as you pivot forward on your right leg and gouge your attacker's eyes with your right hand. This pivot also adds a body defense by turning your neck away from the attacker's grasp. Follow up with a straight knee to the groin with your right leg. Your base leg will probably slide a bit (*glicha*) to accommodate your straight knee to the attacker's groin. If the opponent's groin is too far away for a knee strike, simply extend

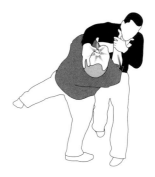

your lower leg, making contact with any part of your lower leg. Follow up with additional *retzev* counterattacks.

Front Collar Choke Defense 2

Tuck your chin and cup both of your hands in front of your face. Curl your fingers in and together to make two hooks with your hands. To remove an attacker's hands from your collar or reduce the choking pressure, use an outward plucking motion with your hands just below the attacker's thumb joint. Do not actually pluck the thumbs. Rather, with a clawlike grip, pluck underneath the thumb where the thumb joint meets the hand. Rest your hands (and your attacker's hands) at the top of your chest muscles. By trapping the attacker's hands against your upper chest just below your clavicle, you eliminate the threat of another attack from his hands. Add a front knee and you have your front choke defense. Follow up with multiple knees, elbows, gouges, and other *retzev* counterattacks.

Note: A variation of this technique is to pluck and clear the choke with a horizontal cross elbow, followed by retzev *combatives.*

Nelson Hold Releases

The half nelson and full nelson wrestling-type holds are used for controlling an opponent. The nelson holds involve an opponent thrusting both of his arms under your armpits from behind (only one arm for the half nelson) and clasping them with a strong grip at the base of your neck. A proper hold never interlaces the fingers. Several variations of these strong holds exist.

Nelson Weight Drop Release

Common sense dictates that the easiest and best defense against the nelson holds is to prevent an opponent from positioning himself behind you.

The most instinctive defense against the nelson hold is dropping your weight and stiffening your shoulders and arms to prevent the attacker from securing his arms behind your neck. To drop your weight, sink your hips by slightly bending your knees and widening your stance. From this position you can use your rear bear hug defense.

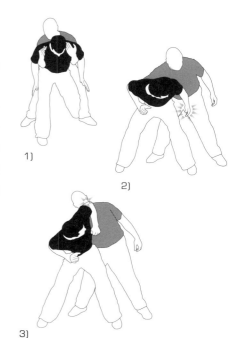

1)

2)

3)

Nelson Clampdown Sidestep Release

This defense allows you to defeat an attacker who is applying a nelson-type hold and pulling you backward. Use the attacker's momentum against him to push him backward off his feet and to land full force on him, followed by retzev *combatives.*

If the defender succeeds in acquiring the hold and tries to take you backward, clamp down on both of the attacker's arms, dropping your weight. Then quickly step to one side and put your leg closest to the attacker behind his closest leg. Step to whichever side of your opponent feels most comfortable to you. Once you have stepped behind him, thrust your weight backward, catching his legs on your

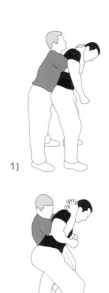

1)

2)

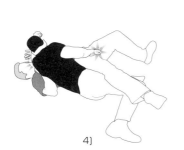

4)

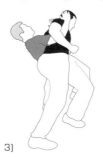

3)

near (inside) leg. As you both fall down make sure to position all of your weight on your attacker's torso. You will crash to the ground, delivering a body blow to his torso with your torso. Finish with rear elbows to the midsection and groin followed by *retzev*.

Hip-Toss Fall Releases

This defense allows you to defeat an attacker who is applying a nelson-type hold and pushing you forward. You will use your powerful hip muscles and the attacker's momentum against him to flip him and turn to land full force on him, followed by retzev *combatives.*

This more advanced technique against an opponent who is driving you forward is to throw the opponent, landing your entire body weight on him and continuing with *retzev*. You will use a basic hip toss with a turn and land on the attacker with all of your weight. The hip toss requires you to square your hips with the attacker's hips or slightly offset your hips in relation to his. Bend your legs slightly and explode up, turning your body to one side. Leverage allows you to throw your attacker by sinking your hips lower than his to jettison him from your back. Lock down on the attacker's arms, and the moment you complete the throw, drop down with the attacker, falling with your full weight on him, followed by *retzev*.

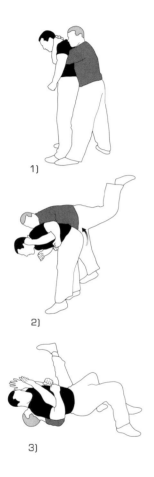

1)

2)

3)

Defensive Throw Against Headlock or Rear Choke with the Attacker Jumping on the Defender

Similar to the nelson hip-toss release, you will jettison your attacker.

This hip toss requires you to square your hips with the attacker's hips or slightly offset your hips. At the same time you must also defend against a headlock or choke by plucking or yanking down on the attacker's arms while tucking your chin. The opponent's arms serve as handles to throw your attacker.

Bend your legs slightly and explode up, turning your body to one side. Leverage again allows you to throw your attacker by sinking your hips lower than his to jettison him from your back. Lock down on the attacker's arms, and the moment you complete the throw, follow with *retzev*. If you fall with the attacker, be sure to drop your weight on him to both increase his impact against the ground and save yourself from the impact.

Advanced Control Defense Against the Rear Bear Hug

This advanced control defense involves placing a control hold lock on the attacker's arm.

If an attacker grabs you from behind with your arms left free, insert your left leg inside the attacker's left leg. You may also wrap your leg around the outside of your opponent's left leg. Inserting or wrapping the leg prevents an assailant from throwing or suplexing you by securing your body to his. After executing your release with rear elbows and an uppercut kick with your heel (not depicted), you will grasp the attacker's left (in this case top-side) wrist with your right hand (you are reaching across your body to secure his left (top) hand, which is grasping the wrist of his right arm.) Secure the attacker's lower hand while turning to the left and snaking your left arm over the top of his left elbow. Take the wrist of his right hand and apply inward pressure to press his elbow firmly to your body. Grab your own opposite wrist to help secure the lock. Squeeze down on his shoulder to apply the control hold (control hold 2). Additional *retzev* combatives can be used if necessary, such as a knee to the groin or head.

Note: You could also insert your right leg inside of the attacker's right leg and perform the mirror opposite technique controlling his right arm and shoulder.

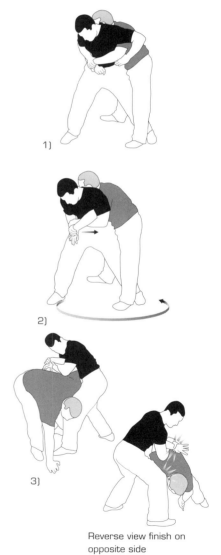

1)

2)

3)

Reverse view finish on opposite side

Defense Against Rear Bear Hug and Being Driven Forward

This defense is similar to the defense against a rear nelson hold when your assailant is driving you forward with your arms free. A bear hug from the rear, also known as a rear clinch, places you in great danger of being driven forward into a wall or the ground or being thrown. The defense is similar to the hip-toss nelson release previously examined. If your arms are free, you will clasp the opponent's arms from over the top to secure his body against yours and use your powerful hip muscles and his momentum to throw him and land full force on top of him. If your arms are pinned, bend them up and use your hips and the attacker's momentum against him to flip him and land full force on to him, followed by retzev combatives.

Regardless of whether your arms are free or pinned, you will use a basic hip toss with a turn and land on the attacker with all of your weight. You will lock down on the attacker's arms and use a modified hip throw while turning your body to drop the attacker backward, with your full weight falling on the attacker. You must keep the attacker close while pinning his arms. Bend your knees and explode up to spin and land on top of the attacker, followed by additional *retzev* counterattacks

Defense Against Front Bear Hug with the Arms Free and Being Driven Back

This highly effective defense involves torquing the attacker's neck using a 180-degree body turn (tsai-bake), placing enormous pressure on the opponent's neck as you use your turning hips and body weight against the opponent's neck while securing one of his legs with your own leg. This is otherwise known as a neck crank.

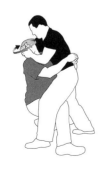

Shoot your hips back slightly and turn your body to the side. This movement creates a stronger body position to resist the push while positioning you to attack the opponent's head. Simultaneously hook your front leg around his same-side leg to secure

your positioning while reaching around his face to embed a finger in his eye or hook under his nose and secure your other hand against his chin. Depending on the attacker's method, his head can be cranked in either direction. You can put tremendous stress on his neck by taking the front leg back 180 degrees to the rear using a *tsai-bake* movement while pushing with the near-side hand and pulling with the far-side hand. Be sure not to take him down and stand over him with his legs between yours, exposing your groin to kicks. A good follow-up after stepping over your downed opponent is a kick to his head with your heel.

Boxing Defense Against Double Leg Takedown

This defense uses footwork and straight punches to the jaw, neck, and ear to defeat an attempt to take you to the ground.

If you do not have time to launch a straight offensive kick or knee to the face of an attacker set on taking you down, a body defense moving off the line using short *tsai-bake* coupled with multiple straight punches can be highly effective. You must execute a strong combination of straight punches to the opponent's jaw and neck, beginning with your near-side arm. You can also jam the attacker with a double palm heel to the head with one hand on the back of the other combined with *tsai-bake*. Follow up with additional *retzev* combatives. Keep in mind that a skilled attacker will not telegraph his intent to take you to the ground. Rather, he will disguise his plan by using combatives or feints against you to shoot when you appear vulnerable.

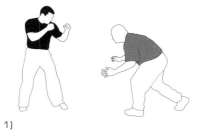

1)

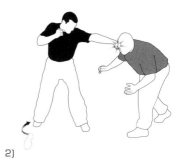

2)

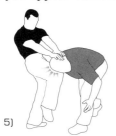

5)

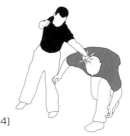

4)

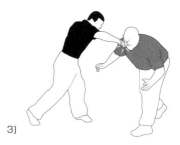

3)

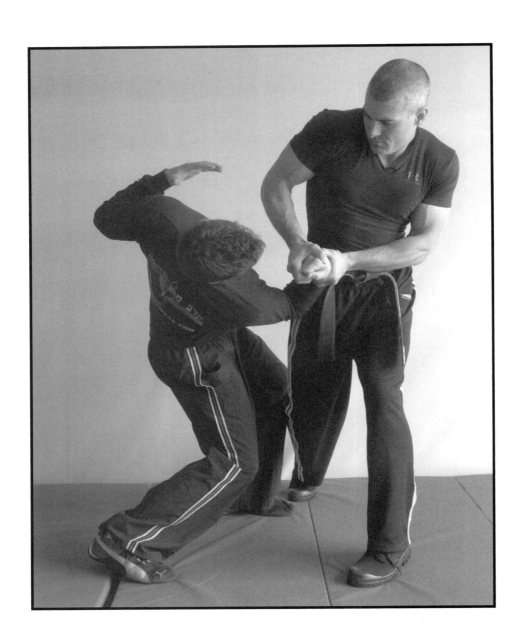

CHAPTER 6

Mastering Infighting, Clinches, Holds, and Takedowns

If long-range lower-body strikes and intermediate-range upper-body strikes do not neutralize your opponent or at least keep him at bay, he can close the distance to grab hold of you. The fight then becomes an "infight," involving short combatives including elbows, knees, uppercut and shovel punches, clinches, and holds. Striking is integral to clinching and other standing control holds, including surprise attacks. To strike, you must create separation from your opponent.

Clinching can be thought of broadly as any control grasp on an opponent's body while both opponents are still standing. Clinching can also involve compact powerful strikes and control holds when two opponents are standing in close proximity. Certain types of clinches are also referred to in defensive *krav maga* vernacular as "bear hugs." In this chapter, you'll learn many infighting techniques and defenses. They all rely on the same principles: always fight back by attacking the weakest points of your opponent's anatomy and using his momentum against him.

Striking in a clinch is different from striking from a distance. In a clinch, body contact can be used to control your opponent. This is especially relevant when an opponent goes to the ground and no longer has the upright support of his legs. Therefore, body contact dictates your fight strategy. In fighting, it is common for one or both opponents to lose balance as a result of tactics or chance, so you need to be prepared for that eventuality.

Once your attacker closes on you, he can attempt life-threatening choke holds, throws, strikes, and neck manipulations. Other types of close-contact grappling include hair pulling, headlocks, and bear hugs, all of which can put you in an extremely exposed position and against which *krav maga* provides defenses. If your attacker manages to work his arms around your torso and begins to throw you, *krav maga* offers powerful instinctive defenses. Advancing your knowledge in such defensive techniques is indispensable.

Getting your opponent off balance is key to close-quarters infighting. Do this by setting up *retzev* combatives including strikes, throws, and joint locks. Wherever the head goes, the body will follow. Taking an opponent off balance leads to other *retzev* combative techniques because the opponent is concerned not only with protecting himself but also with recovering his balance. You must take the opponent in a direction he does not expect to go.

Clinching

In a superior clinch position, you can trap your opponent's head and torso, making both attack and defense difficult for your opponent while maintaining your own combative options, primarily elbows, short uppercuts and hook and shovel punches, knee strikes to the groin and midsection (especially switching knees and roundhouse knee shots), locks, chokes, takedowns, and throws. You may, of course, also gouge your opponent's eyes with your thumbs prior to acquiring control of the head.

The clinch can give you several advantages by controlling your opponent's ability to strike you, your position for powerful short devastating combatives, and his attempts to take you down. The last point requires emphasis. The clinch can both save you from being taken down and be used to take your opponent down, depending on how you employ it.

We will focus primarily on the crown-of-the-head and rear clinches, which afford great control over your opponent. These clinches provide the option of strikes and takedowns into superior ground-fighting positions. A third clinching position that is heavily emphasized in the *krav maga* curriculum is the symmetrical clinch.

Crown-of-the-Head Clinch

This powerful combative allows you strong control of your opponent by clasping the top of his skull, setting you up for knees, vertical elbows, guillotine chokes, and neck torquing movements. You may also gouge his eyes with your thumb prior to encircling his head with your arms.

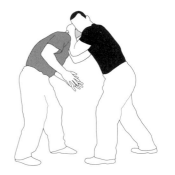

Place one hand on the crown of your opponent's head and your other hand on top of the first. Always vie for inside hand position—both of your arms are inside of your opponent's arms and exerting pressure on the rear crown of his head—to allow better control over the opponent. Try not to grab the base of the neck, and do not interlock your fingers in this (or any other) combative. Squeeze your elbows together, forcing your opponent's head to your chest level to further throw him off balance.

Keep your opponent's head lower than your own and pressed into your chest; do not allow separation. The head clinch places your adversary in a vulnerable position for knee strikes, vertical elbows, guillotine chokes, and neck torquing movements. To defend against this type of clinch, we would target the groin, so your opponent might do the same to you—one of the drawbacks to this technique.

This clinch may also be used to defend against an opponent wrapping his arms around your waist under your arms (a bear hug). Simply apply the clinch and shoot both of your legs back to create separation. Knee strikes and other *retzev* combatives become readily available from this position.

Clinch Canting Opponent's Neck

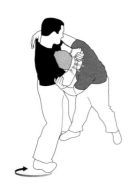

This clinch variation gives you the ability to take your opponent down with severe torquing pressure on the neck, known as a neck crank.

From the inside clinch position, you will change your grip by clasping one hand with the other as though you are wringing your hands. Your forearms will now make contact with the neck. You will then use your upper forearm to twist the neck of your opponent and pull the side of his face to your chest. Complete the move with a 180-degree circle step (*tsai-bake*). When squeezing your elbows together, it is best to position one of your forearms slightly ahead of the other to force your opponent's head into an awkward angle, causing him discomfort and throwing him off balance. For further effect, yank his head sharply toward you or from side to side using your forearms and chest as a vise. This variation also allows for a takedown by performing the *tsai-bake* footwork we will discuss for Cavalier 1. This uses all of your body weight to torque him down by the neck. In other words, if you have your opponent in this clinch with your right hand on top (his face is pointed to your left), you will move your leg in a semicircle to take him down. Another option is simply to snap the opponent's head forward while stepping back with your front leg for added torque and power.

Clinch Transition to Neck Crank

This easy yet powerful transition gives you another tool to take your opponent down.

After securing the crown-of-the-head clinch, you will remove your right hand and bring it quickly to your opponent's chin. You will force your opponent's chin sideways to the left while releasing your left arm to secure your opponent's forehead or right eye socket. Torque or crank his neck to the side using a *tsai-bake* movement with the left leg.

Rear Body Clinch

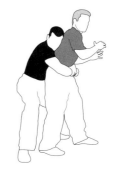

The rear clinch allows you to position yourself behind your opponent for control and takedowns.

Your grip can vary, but I prefer grabbing my forearm with my other hand for a tight hold, as depicted. Another strong hold is to clasp your hands together as if you were clapping, with the thumbs pressed against the hands. You must keep your head properly positioned and close to your opponent's back. Remember, *krav maga* defenses utilize rear horizontal elbows against a rear bear hug, so watch for this counterstrike.

Symmetrical Head Clinch

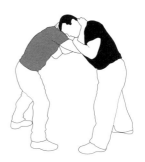

The symmetrical clinch is when two fighters lock up with each other with one hand behind the opponent's head and the other locked securely in the crook of his elbow. Neither fighter has a decisive advantage.

Your left arm is wrapped around the crook of your opponent's right elbow or upper arm, with your right arm around his head. He is doing the same to you. Your head is positioned on the side of your arm hooking the opponent's head. This position gives neither one of you an advantage. What you can do to him, he can

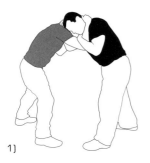

1)

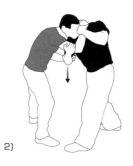

2)

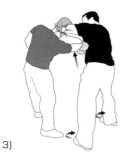

3)

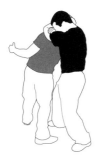

4)

do to you. Think this through. *Krav maga* provides options that can take your opponent off guard:

- If your opponent grabs you around the waist, defend by using the crown-of-the head clinch or clinch cant variation while creating separation by shooting your legs back or sprawling.
- From the symmetrical clinch, reach across with your right arm to cross-grab the opponent's right clinched elbow from underneath while turning his body to your right and delivering a horizontal left elbow or reaching around the opponent's face for a neck crank, face bar takedown, choke, or shredding the face with your fingers. Another option is to reach across with your right arm to the inside to push away the opponent's right clinched arm and deliver a horizontal left elbow.
- Neutralize your opponent (while in clinch) by cross-grabbing the opponent's elbow at the crook, yanking down, and coming over the top with a horizontal or inverted elbow followed by additional combatives.
- From the symmetrical clinch, remove your hand from behind his head to gouge his eye and then deliver a horizontal elbow strike.
- Yank his head down into a standing guillotine choke hold.

HEAD CLINCH DRILL

From a crown-of-the-head or symmetrical clinch, the snaking drill allows you and a partner to vie for inside position. As noted, in a crown-of-the-head clinch, inside position strategically locates both of your arms inside your opponent's arms. For the drill, one partner applies the crown-of-the-head clinch. The other partner inserts one arm and then the other inside the clinching partner's arms to achieve inside position. Do not insert both arms at the same time. Then the partner who was displaced from the superior inside position snakes his arms (one at a time) to reacquire the position. You should trade positions in one-minute intervals. Be careful not to damage your partner's ears.

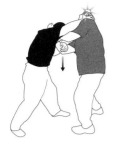

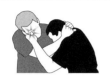

Defenses Against the Clinch

The clinch can place you in a precarious position susceptible to devastating knee, elbow, and neck manipulations, so it is imperative to defend yourself if your opponent takes you into the clinch.

A simple defense is to attack your opponent's eyes with a thumb gouge. You should be able to access his eye socket even if he buries his head. Another defense is to reach across and yank down underneath one arm, keeping your elbow tip down to defend against knee strikes. Deliver a horizontal elbow with your other arm to the rear of the attacker's head. A variation of this defense is to reach across and disengage the attacker's arm with a push followed by a horizontal elbow strike with your free arm to the rear of the attacker's head or to apply a rear choke. A final option is to push up on the opponent's other arm while lowering your center of gravity to slip under the clinch with simultaneous strikes to the groin. Note, however, that this can be difficult against a strong and technically skilled opponent.

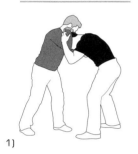

1)

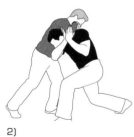

2)

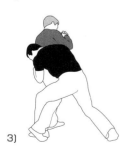

3)

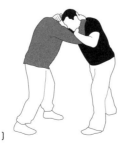

1)

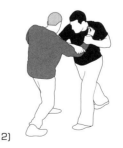

2)

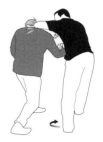

3)

The Standing Guillotine Hold

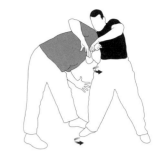

The standing guillotine hold, if properly applied, is a fight ender. It provides you with a multifaceted attack: you can exert a standing choke, strike with your knees, and take him down (with the option of a pincered guillotine choke or neck crank). Your opponent has few defensive options. When you add combatives such as a straight knee to the groin that can force his head to sink below yours if he attacks your legs with a takedown, or you can transition from this hold to the neck clinch.

Trap your opponent's head and one of his arms by wrapping your arm around his neck and inserting your other arm to exert control or choking pressure against his windpipe. Your grip can vary, but clasping the hands is usually preferred. Keep your elbows in. Depending on how your opponent reacts, this hold can also result in a blood choke. You can also push against the shoulder of your opponent with your non-locked arm while clasping your pushing forearm to extend his neck for a deeper choke.

Trap Against Opponent's Lead Arm with Over-the-Top Punch or Elbow

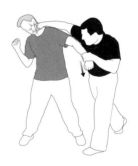

This offensive technique is useful in catching your opponent unaware in the beginning stages of a fight. You will trap your opponent's lead arm while delivering a simultaneous over-the-top elbow to the opponent's temple or straight punch to the opponent's throat followed by retzev *combatives.*

Adjusting your body position slightly to the outside of the opponent's lead arm, you will trap his lead arm by turning your lead wrist in and clamping down on your opponent's lead arm to defeat his defense against your simultaneous over-the-top punch or elbow.

Head Butts and Defenses Against Head Butts

A strong neck allows for the head to be used as a valuable personal weapon. Head butts can have a debilitating effect on an opponent, often taking an adversary by surprise, especially when infighting. Primary targets on an opponent include the nose, eye socket, and ear. The strike is optimally delivered with the front of the crown of the head or the thickest frontal area of the forehead. The back of the head may also be used with devastating effect against an opponent behind you. (Note that the temple is the thinnest part of the skull, while the upper part of the forehead is the thickest.) Keep in mind that making your head a battering ram is not necessarily a wise option. Nevertheless, it has its place in your arsenal.

The Front and Rear Head Butts

The head butt uses the crown of the skull to target the opponent's nose or eyebrow ridges. This technique can be especially effective when taking an opponent by surprise by sinking your head into your shoulders to use your whole body as a battering ram.

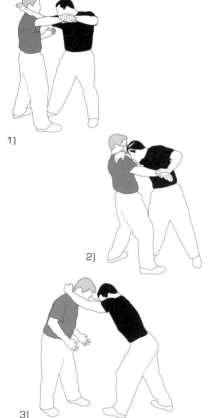

1)

2)

3)

To prepare for a head butt, you must bull your neck, keep your tongue free of your teeth, and strengthen your jaw by keeping space between your upper and lower teeth. Your entire body is behind the strike, not just your neck muscles. Power comes from the torso rather than just the neck, along with your entire body moving through the strike. A rear head butt option is also available using a similar technique against the opponent's nose or brow ridge. The head butt is not suitable for everyone. Note that the technique should not use crown of the head against crown of the head.

Two head butt variations are illustrated: one from the crown-

of-the-head clinch (covered in this chapter) and one with a forearm brace (an offensive movement by itself) across the opponent's
throat. This provides you with the ability to head-butt but safe-
guards you against an opponent attempting to head-butt you.

The rear head butt is highly effective against someone grabbing you from behind. As with the front head butt, your principal
targets are the opponent's nose and brow ridge. Your entire body
delivers the strike by bulling your shoulders and moving from
the waist; do not strike only with your head.

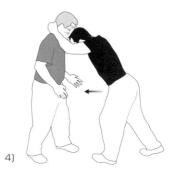

4]

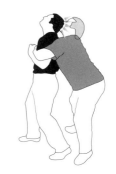

Defense Against Head Butts

*A simple raised elbow parallel to the ground is a formidable deterrent to
your opponent delivering a head butt. It also provides you with the ability to strike. You may also clear the attacker's arms with a horizontal elbow strike, as shown in chapter 8.*

Raise your elbow with your triceps parallel to the ground to
block and simultaneously deliver a blow to your opponent's incoming head.

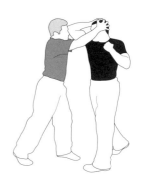

Takedowns

Krav maga incorporates several types of opponent takedowns, including sweeps, cavaliers, control holds, and throws.

CAVALIERS

Cavaliers are designed to use your powerful hip muscles and body weight torque against an opponent's wrist to take him down. There are two types of cavaliers frequently used in *krav maga*. Cavaliers are usually preceded by *retzev* combatives to soften up the opponent. If you meet resistance, you may distract your opponent with a kick to the shin or a knee to the thigh to facilitate compliance. These softeners can be escalated into full-force strikes to the groin or punches to the neck. The following cavalier can also be modified for weapons takedown and removal.

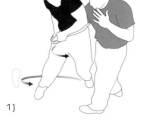

1)

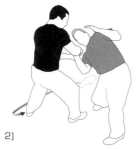

2)

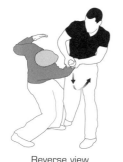

Reverse view

The Cavalier

This powerful takedown places enormous pressure on an opponent's wrist, forcing him down to the ground. You can follow up with a strong kick to the head, midsection, or groin along with an arm bar. This takedown is a logical follow-up to the inside 90-degree block defense you learned in chapter 2.

The Cavalier secures your opponent's right hand when you are positioned behind his right shoulder and to his side. If you are securing your opponent's right hand for the takedown, you will place your right hand on top of his right hand, knuckles to knuckles. Your left hand will then secure his right forearm just below the wrist. Do not grab the wrist, as this will hinder your desired objective of applying maximum torquing pressure to the wrist. The wrist is flexible, but not when simultaneous inward and side pressure is applied. If you encounter a strong opponent, you may loosen him up by using a knee or other combative, including a vertical uppercut elbow to the back of his clenched fist. These strikes both distract and physically undermine your opponent's ability to resist. To apply the torquing pressure, you will take a 180-degree rear step with your left leg (*tsai-bake*). Once you have taken your opponent down, do not let go of the wrist. Rather, keep applying upward pressure to keep his right shoulder off the ground. Many offensive combatives can be used at this point, such as a heel stomp to your attacker or a scissors arm bar that will break the arm. You may also use this control hold to rotate an opponent on his stomach to apply a facedown control hold.

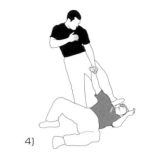
4)

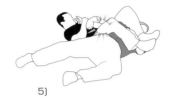
5)

Note: One variation of this takedown places both of your thumbs to the back of the opponent's hand to put downward pressure on the wrist. Another variation places downward pressure on the wrist with the palm of your same-side hand without clasping the opponent's hand.

For law enforcement and security personnel, once you have taken the opponent down on his back, you may reverse him onto his stomach by yanking up on his arm and stepping 180 degrees in the opposite direction while clipping the arm just below the elbow with your knee to force him to turn onto his stomach. You will be in a strong position to collapse his straight arm for face-down control and the application of restraints.

An advanced variation utilizes a jumping scissors kick to the opponent's groin while applying crushing wrist pressure to the opponent.

The footwork performed in this takedown can easily be applied to a crown-of-the-head clinch takedown as described previously. You must keep the opponent's head tight to your chest to create the necessary control and torque to effectively take him down.

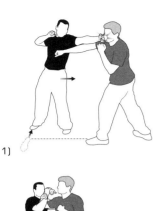

1)

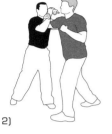

2)

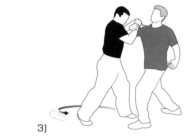

3)

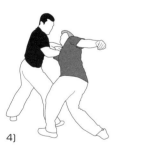

4)

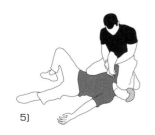

5)

CONTROL HOLDS

Control Hold 1

This highly adaptable control hold allows an attacker to be taken down swiftly backward with strong dead-side positional control.

Control hold 1 may be applied with or without preceding *retzev* combatives. The hold places compliance or takedown pressure on the opponent's shoulder and wrist. If you are facing or positioned to the side of your opponent, you will grab his right wrist with your right hand. Grip the flat of the back of his hand with a perpendicular grip. You can push his face away to cause a distraction. You will curl his wrist in while slipping your other arm just below the shoulder, over the top of his targeted arm, and across his forearm, using a figure-four grip. You will then reach around the arm and encircle it to grip your own forearm, tightening your right arm to your body. Bring his elbow and wrist close to your body, take a 180-degree rear step (*tsai-bake*) with your left leg similar to Cavalier 1, bringing your opponent down. As your opponent is going down, keep the grip tight. Once your opponent is down, you may use an additional knee strike to his head for further compliance or simply rest your knee on his head while exerting pressure on the wrist and shoulder. The opponent may also be rotated onto his stomach.

Note: For law enforcement and security personnel, once you have taken the opponent down on his back, you may reverse him onto his stomach by yanking up on his arm while still maintaining your figure-four grip and turning in the opposite direction. Do not, however, break the movements by touching your knees to the ground. You must maintain the momentum of takedown into an immediate reversal onto his stomach. By keeping strong pressure on his wrist and shoulder to facilitate his turn, you have taken him down by combining a joint lock and a 180-degree step in one direction and now will take a 180-degree step and turn in the opposite direction, turning his wrist and shoulder in the opposite direction that you initially turned to take him down. You will be in a strong position to apply restraints and control his movement.

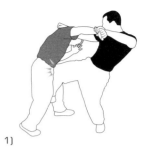
1)

Control Hold 2

This highly practical and effective control hold allows an attacker to be taken down swiftly with strong dead-side positional control and driven face first into the ground.

Control hold 2 may be applied with or without preceding *retzev* combatives. The hold places compliance or takedown pressure on the opponent's wrist and shoulder. If you are facing your opponent or the side of your opponent, you will grab his right wrist with your left hand. Another option is to grip the flat of the back of his hand by turning your wrist up to create pressure on his wrist. You will raise your wrist, placing upward pressure, so that his arm comes up with a 90-degree bend with fingers toward the ground. Reach over the top of his targeted shoulder, clamping down hard on the shoulder while snaking your right arm over the top of his targeted arm and across his shoulder to clasp your other arm. It is imperative that you clamp down on the shoulder to facilitate the lock. You will then reach around the arm and encircle it to grip your own forearm. Bring his elbow and wrist close to your body, keeping hard pressure on the shoulder. Take a 180-degree step with your right leg to bring down your opponent. As your opponent is going down, keep the grip tight. You may further secure him by placing your right knee behind his elbow, exerting upward pressure on the shoulder, and your left knee on top of his neck.

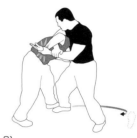
2)

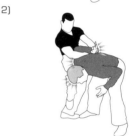
Variation with knee combatives

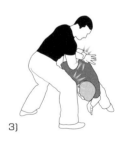
3)

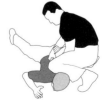
Opposite arm finish view

TRUE KRAVIST

Times Square, New York, in Rich's Own Words

A few weeks after starting *krav maga* training and a day after we had done control holds and takedowns, we had an incident at the restaurant I managed in Times Square. In the middle of happy hour we had trouble with two large patrons. They became rude and were asked to leave. They tried to leave the restaurant without paying their bill. The conversation spilled into the middle of Forty-second Street. I was the smallest of the group of six managers and considerably smaller then the two patrons. We called the police, but they were slow to arrive because of shift change and heavy traffic. We cornered the two bill dodgers, but one guy split. I followed him along the crowded sidewalk while wearing cook's clothing. As I pursued the guy, he stopped and bent over to take a weapon out of his sock. I immediately squared off for a rear leg kick to his head. He saw my intent and started to run rather than retrieve his weapon. While yelling for the police, I tackled the guy and put him in a control hold I had just learned in the training. The first cop on scene said, "Nice takedown. Are you a cop or security?" I said, "No, I'm a kitchen manager who takes *krav maga*"—which has always served me well.

Three Body Takedowns

There are more than two dozen takedowns and throws in the first three levels of *krav maga*. The following are three of the most elementary and utilitarian techniques.

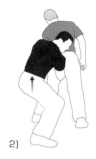

Bucket Scoop Takedown

This extremely potent takedown allows you to strike the opponent's groin from the rear while dropping him facedown onto the ground. This technique can be used as a follow-up to many techniques, including an outside block against a hook or the sliding punch defense you learned in chapter 2. While not illustrated, this technique may also be used as a frontal combative when facing an opponent to slam him down to the ground with your body weight on top of him.

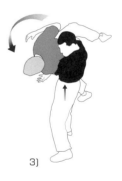

The bucket scoop takes you to your opponent's dead side, optimally pinning his closest arm to you with your left arm and shoulder while slamming your right forearm between his legs. As you strike or grab his testicles, position your hips slightly behind him to throw him on his head. Pinning his arm will hinder his ability to cushion his fall. You must sink your hips into your opponent and keep your back straight. As with all throws, power emanates from your hips and core. Explode up, keeping your back straight and head tucked to avoid an elbow counterstrike from his free arm. The throwing motion loosely resembles pouring out a bucket, hence the name.

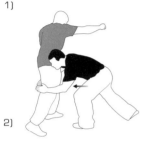

1)

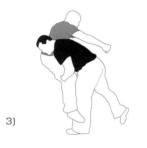

2)

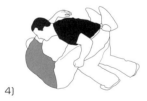

3)

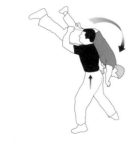

4)

5) Variation of double leg takedown

Double Leg Takedown Tackle

The tackle takedown is designed to put your opponent on his back with you in a strong position to continue retzev *counterattacks.*

The tackle is one of the most effective takedown techniques and should be set up with previous combatives or a feint, usually a punch or head strike. Like other combatives, the tackle's power derives from hip and leg explosion. Your attack point should be driving your shoulder just below your opponent's hips or midsection with your head to one side of his torso. You should bull your neck and keep your face up. Usually from a short running start, and just prior to contact, you will sink your hips with a wide leg base to explode through your opponent, similar to rising from a squat but also churning your legs for momentum. Optimally, you will wrap your arms around your opponent's legs at the knees to buckle them. You may land with one of your knees smashing into the opponent's groin or quickly transition into a high mount, discussed in chapter 7. To be sure, the tackle is not a suitable technique for everyone because of strength and size considerations. The technique can be especially effective when combined with a roll to defend against certain types of attacks such as an opponent threatening with a chain twirling around his head. Two variations include picking your opponent up and slamming him to the ground, by either tossing him over your shoulder or body-slamming him to the ground.

The double leg takedown takes your opponent to the ground but differs in the execution and your position with respect to the opponent. As with a conventional tackle, the double leg takedown is best executed by setting the technique up with previous combatives or a feint. You must be careful when executing this technique not to take a kick or knee to the head; stay out of the line of fire. Note that a kick or knee to the head is one of *krav maga's* preferred timing defenses to defeat a double leg takedown. A timing defense involves a preemptive combative to stop the opponent before he initiates or as he initiates his attack. To initiate the double leg takedown from the left outlet stance, you will aim at the opponent's left leg (he is also in a left outlet stance). Keeping your head tucked, you will dip down, bending your left knee and aiming it between the opponent's legs. Your right leg will dip down (similar to performing a modified lunge) while your left leg gently glides to the ground. Do not slam your left knee into the ground full force. As with the tackle, you will drive your right shoulder into your opponent, but this time at thigh level, keeping your head to the side of his right hip. Encircle your opponent's legs with your arms at the back of his knees. Yank his legs forward into you, buckling his knees. Proceed with groin strikes and *retzev* combatives. This position is easily transitioned into the mount examined in chapter 6. You may also throw your opponent over your shoulders facedown or body-slam him into the ground—both devastating variations.

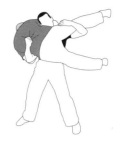

Variation of double leg takedown into a body slam

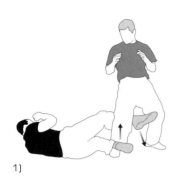

1)

Scissors Leg Takedown

A useful takedown from the ground is catching your opponent's legs in a scissoring action that will put your opponent down flat on his face, setting him up for a withering array of additional combatives. There are two options for this takedown: either scissoring to the rear with your top leg (as depicted) or scissoring forward with your top leg when facing in the opposite direction.

If you find yourself on the ground and on your side, you can take your opponent down by catching your opponent with your leg touching the ground at his ankle and scissoring his leg with your other leg by delivering a horizontal reverse leg kick. A leg lock (examined in chapter 6) with a choke is a good follow-up option to facilitate your *retzev* counterattack.

Another takedown is a side kick to the kneecap while scissoring your dead-side leg behind his heel with devastating effect.

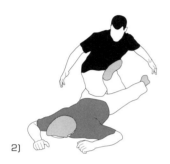

2)

Note: A "flying" version of this reverse scissors technique may also be used while you and your opponent are still standing, but this requires exquisite timing.

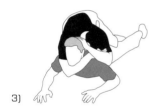

3)

COMBINATION TECHNIQUE: HOOK PUNCH
DEFENSE WITH SPIN INTO CHOKE

This technique demonstrates the continuous combat flow of *krav maga* by defending one of the most common attacks, a hook punch. You will simultaneously block and attack using a straight punch, web strike to the throat, palm heel, or other option. Maintain contact with your blocking arm and reach underneath the opponent's elbow to secure it just below the crook with a cupped hook keeping your thumb aligned with your hand. Reach underneath his elbow and pull your opponent back to you with both hands, using *tsai-bake* footwork to spin his torso and put his back to you. Execute the choke (which you will perfect in chapter 7). Other follow-up options include ripping and tearing the attacker's face by inserting fingers (fishhooks) into your opponent's eyes and clawing the face and throat. You may also clinch the face from the rear to sprawl your opponent backward with the option of a knee to the base of the skull or spine.

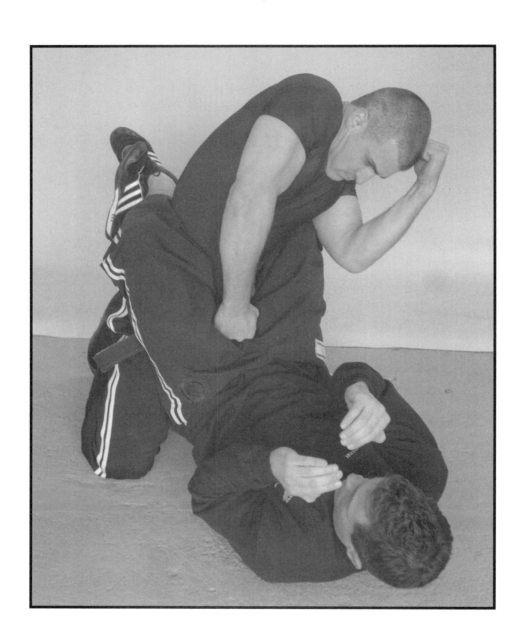

CHAPTER 7

Groundwork

Israeli *krav maga* groundwork can generally be summarized as "what we do up, we do down." In other words, in *krav maga*, whatever we do from an upright position, we do from a ground position, with modifications and with weight properly positioned. Just as there are no rules in an "up" fight, there are no rules in a "down" fight. Groin strikes, throat strikes, eye gouges, and biting all are viable ground-fighting options. Beginning in the early 1990s, Grandmaster Haim Gidon began to revamp the *krav maga* curriculum, adding extensive groundwork approved by Imi, who sat in Haim's gym monitoring, mentoring, and enjoying the continuing evolution of *krav maga*.

Importantly, you should always try to stay on your feet. While on the ground you are vulnerable to additional attackers, and environmental hazards such as broken glass.

Krav maga ground techniques incorporate both defensive and offensive tactics. In this book, we will examine only a few of the core techniques. Several volumes could be written on the Israeli system's ground-fighting capabilities. As of the date of this writing, in orange belt alone (the second belt level) there are more than fifty joint and neck lock and choke variations. In green belt (the third belt level) there are more than eighty-five ground combative variations. Blue belt (the fourth belt level), brown belt (the fifth belt level), and advanced successive black belts (the sixth level and higher) each add techniques at cumulative and correspondingly comprehensive levels. Nevertheless, with each advanced belt level, the basics form the building blocks.

Arm Bars and Shoulder Dislocations

The arms and hands are the most flexible parts of the body with the greatest ranges of motion. Structurally, the elbow is the weakest part of the arm. An opponent's elbow position will either be bent or straight. Plan your counterattack accordingly. The shoulder joint is the upper body's largest joint and has a ball-and-socket operating mechanism. The joint's head (ball) is much larger than the socket anchoring it to the body. It is held in place by relatively weak ligaments, making it highly susceptible to dislocation.

The elbow joint is composed of three mutually supportive joints. The elbow's rotation is controlled by the shoulder joint. Locking the wrist will lock the elbow, which in turn will lock the shoulder. Therefore, controlling the elbow and locking the shoulder allows for the most highly effective wrist locks. Optimally, in a ground fight you can lock the opponent's joints in unison. While a single joint lock can be effective, it may still allow your opponent the opportunity for counterattack.

Attacks to the Neck

Protecting your head, neck, and spine during a confrontation is vital. The ability to defend against choke and neck manipulations is paramount in all aspects of a fight, particularly the ground phase. A broken neck or spine can paralyze or kill. Hair may be used to torque the neck, exposing the throat to attack. To yank the head back you need to grasp the front of the scalp, running your fingers through the hair and making a tight fist to increase the leverage of the pull. Closely cropped hair or no hair provides an advantage to guard against such neck manipulations.

Counterattacks to the head and neck can shut the body down temporarily or permanently. The neck is extremely vulnerable because of its vital air passages, arteries, and nerves that sustain proper brain function. The spinal column at the base of the neck is highly susceptible to injury from strikes, throws and locks, with potentially lethal consequences if the spinal nerves are severed. Striking, manipulating, and twisting the neck can injure the arteries and vertebrae. In a defensive mode, you must take great care to protect these vital areas through proper technique and body positioning. *Chokes are a quick fight ender*. You must not allow anyone to get their hand, arms, or legs around your neck.

Animals immediately attack the throat as the most efficient method to bring down their prey, and trained street fighters do the same. Techniques that force the head forward, back, or sideways can produce serious injury to the neck, specifically the cervical vertebrae. The key to executing proper chokes is using your hands and arms to provide leverage and compression against an opponent, leaving your opponent few, if any, defenses. The narrower the choking implement, the easier the penetration of the opponent's neck. The ulnar and radial edges of the wrist and forearm are particularly well suited to apply compression to the throat and neck. An opponent's clothing can be readily used to choke him—and, correspondingly, so can yours, so beware.

Protecting your throat and neck is vital. Tucking your chin and keeping your shoulders lifted is a necessary and immediate defense against an attack to the neck; however, these are only preliminary measures. They can easily be defeated by an attacker who yanks your hair back or applies pressure against your philtrum, eye sockets, or other pressure points.

Dead-Side and Positional Control

Once you are committed to a fight, your goal is to put yourself in a dominant position. Never turn your back to your opponent in any type of fight situation, especially if this puts you facedown on the ground, the worst possible position. From this position the back of your head and neck are exposed to attack. Nearly as dangerous is if the opponent secures you from behind or "takes your back" with his legs pincered around your torso or a body triangle clamp where he folds one leg under a knee, creating a figure four. As with dead-side position in a standing fight, optimally you will achieve a side-mount or rear-mount position in a ground fight. There are four preferred *krav maga* ground positions: rear mount, side straddle knee or stomach, side mount chest down, and high mount while controlling the opponent's arms. Punishing combatives, joint break locks, and choke options are readily available from these positions.

Krav maga rarely relies on joint break locks and chokes without first engaging in *retzev* combative attacks. Think of it as softening up your opponent. An opponent defending against combative strikes may put himself in a vulnerable position for joint break locks and chokes. Many fighters rely heavily on the hands for combatives and the feet primarily for movement. Keep in mind that in a ground fight the legs become highly important for gaining control over an opponent or kick combatives when your back is on the ground. To achieve a lock, it is paramount that you keep your hips close to your opponent's targeted joint. Positional control is crucial. Ease of transition or ground *retzev* must be second nature.

The following table is an overview of your most and least advantageous positions with respect to an opponent. These five basic positions specifically take into account groin, throat, and neck strikes and your ability to defend against an opponent using these same attacks.

The positions you *most* want to be in	The positions you *least* want to be in
1. You are straddling your opponent from behind while he is face down with your legs hooked into his sides—the rear-mount position.	1. You are facedown with your opponent straddling you from behind with his legs hooked into your sides—the rear-mount position.
2. You are behind your opponent with your legs pincered around him but not crossed at the ankles, or one leg is placed parallel across his midsection while the other leg hooks the ankle and clamps down to form a figure-four lock.	2. Your opponent is behind you and has his legs pincered around you but not crossed at the ankles or one leg is placed parallel across your mid-section while the other leg hooks the ankle and clamps down to form a figure-four lock. Alternatively, you are facedown, resting on your elbows and knees, covering your head with your hands (the "turtle position").
3. You are mounted high on your opponent, trapping his arms and keeping his back flat to the ground, limiting his escape options.	3. Your opponent is mounted high on you and has trapped your arms with your back flat to the ground, limiting your escape options,
4. You are side-mounted on your opponent, controlling his arms, or have a knee-on-stomach mount with control of the opponent's nearside arm.	4. Your opponent is side-mounted on you, controlling your arms, or has you in a knee-on-stomach position, controlling your near-side arm.
5. You have side control of your opponent chest down.	5. Your opponent has side control of you chest down.

A Note on the Mount and High Closed Guard Positions

The mount (where you are straddling your opponent with his back to the ground and your heels are hooked underneath his rib cage) and the high closed guard (where your back is to the ground and your opponent is pincered between your legs, which are hooked at the ankles) are well-known and formidable fighting positions. There should be little doubt of their proven efficacy in the ring. Yet there is one crucial streetfighting vulnerability if your opponent maintains proper position: your groin, throat, and eyes are susceptible to attack. Further clarified:

- If Fighter 1 (F1) achieves the mount, unless he rides high and traps his opponent's arms, his groin is highly vulnerable to hand and elbow strikes by Fighter 2 (F2), who is underneath F1.
- When in the high closed guard, if F2 maintains correct posture and position (his opponent does not control his arms and upper body), he can attack F1's groin using hand and elbow strikes even if F1 rides him hard with his closed guard. Knees to the groin and coccyx are also potential vulnerabilities.

Professional no-holds-barred fighters are some of the toughest, most athletic, best-conditioned, and most highly skilled athletes in the world. In the sports arena, these great professional fighters face mandatory target restrictions for organized fighting, including no groin, throat, eye, kidney, or spine attacks. As you now know, these debilitating attacks can maim an attacker and end a fight quickly. What these pro fighters are barred from doing is precisely what you must do. In other words, these targets combined with other vulnerable areas are your priority targets.

CHEST DOWN BODY POSITIONING DRILL

Body positioning is the core of groundwork. This yellow-belt drill will familiarize you with the body positions.

One partner lies flat faceup with hands at the side while the other partner plants his chest on the his partner's. The partner on top will use the palms of his hands and balls of his feet to perform a 360-degree circle with his weight bearing down on the stationary partner's chest while keeping him pinned flush to the ground. This drill will begin to make you comfortable with all of the body positions on the ground from both the top (when you do the drill with your partner) and from the bottom (when the partner does the drill with you.) Note that as a defender, you never should have your back flat on the ground because of the lack of mobility.

Releases and Defenses

Of course, the best release and defense against locks, either while standing or on the ground, is to avoid putting yourself in the vulnerable position in the first place. As noted, chokes and joint lock breaks are fight enders. While you can use them with great efficiency, remember that they can be used against you. Keeping your chin tucked and limbs safe is key. This preemptive body positioning cannot be overemphasized. The following sections are ordered by the best body position advantage to you against an opponent, as referred to in the previous grid.

OFFENSES FROM THE REAR MOUNT

When taking the opponent's back or positioning your chest to his back with his torso between your legs—the most advantageous position—you have an array of combative strikes at your disposal in addition to chokes, including elbows and forearm strikes to the back of the neck, eye gouges, and heel kicks to your opponent's groin and abdomen.

Chokes

Chokes must only be used in a self-defense situation where you have an acute fear that the attacker intends you serious bodily harm. In *krav maga* parlance, there are two types of choke holds: chokes and blood chokes. Both techniques achieve the same result: unconsciousness, brain damage, or death, depending on the force and length of time the choke is applied.

Chokes cut off the oxygen supply to the brain by preventing air from refilling the lungs. In addition, a choke can cause severe damage to the trachea, hyoid bone, and larynx. (Be aware that a choke or strangulation technique can exacerbate or trigger a pre-existing medical condition, resulting in death.) The tongue can also become lodged in back of the throat, occluding airflow. Blood chokes stop the flow of blood by constricting the carotid artery and jugular veins on the sides of the neck that carry oxygenated and deoxygenated blood.*

Chokes are fight enders. As emphasized, you must not allow anyone to get their hand, arms, or legs around your neck. Tucking your chin and lifting your shoulders are necessary preliminary defenses. These initial defenses, however, can easily be defeated by an attacker who yanks your hair back or applies pressure against

---

*The majority of the blood flowing to the brain is delivered by the carotid arteries. The carotid artery and vagus nerve are positioned under the jugular vein. Usually, unconsciousness will result in as few as seven seconds. Blood chokes are more efficient and inflict less pain on the opponent.

your philtrum, eye sockets, or other susceptible pressure points, forcing you to lift your chin, which exposes your throat.

Choke techniques can utilize the hands, forearm, or objects such as a stick or rolled-up magazine placed across the throat. The key to proper chokes is using your hands and arms to provide leverage and strong compression that leaves your opponent few, if any, defenses. The ulnar and radial edges of the wrist and forearm are particularly well suited to apply compression to the throat and neck. An opponent's clothing can be used against him—and so can yours, so beware. You must keep your head close to your opponent to avoid countertechniques. The following three techniques are applied from the rear; the most advantageous choking position.

You should use three people when practicing choke holds—two to drill and the third to monitor the situation to ensure the person applying the technique stops at the instant the choke is successfully applied or at the first sign of danger. When practicing with a partner you must take the utmost care. When allowing yourself to be choked, you will not be able to speak if the choke is properly applied. So you must have a prearranged signal such as tapping your partner to tell him to immediately release the choke.

Blade of the Forearm Choke

A choke using the blade of the forearm applies crushing pressure to the opponent's windpipe by using the radius or blade of the forearm, depriving his brain of oxygen. This pressure can collapse and crush the windpipe. Keep your body tight to your opponent and tuck your head. Clasp your non-choking arm with your hand and pull your forearm into you. When practicing with a partner use extreme caution.

Crook of the Elbow Choke

A blood choke using the crook of the elbow applies pressure to the opponent's carotid sheath on both sides of the neck, occluding blood flow to his brain. Pressure is applied using your bicep muscle and radius of the arm. Keep your body tight to your opponent with your head tucked. Clasp your right hand with your left hand and squeeze your arm to constrict blood flow. When practicing with a partner you must use extreme caution.

Professional Rear Naked Choke

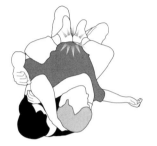

The professional rear naked choke can be thought of as a superior combination of the two previous choking techniques because of the extreme pressure that may be applied. The blade of the forearm and bicep apply pressure to the opponent's carotid sheath on both sides of the neck, stopping blood flow to his brain. You will grab your left biceps with your right hand. The non-choking arm will snake behind your opponent's head and place your hand on the rear of his skull. Do not place the hand too high because a defender can remove it or pluck it away to disable the choke. To apply pressure, squeeze your choking arm toward you and your non-choking arm's biceps while exerting pressure forward with your cupped hand and leaning the side of your head into your hand for added choking pressure. Your body is essentially both leaning forward and then pulling back to exert maximum choking pressure. Keep your body tight to your opponent and tuck your head. Clasp your hand with your non-choking arm and squeeze your arm to constrict blood flow. This choke is highly effective. You should keep your hips square to have the opportunity to apply the choke with either arm. When on the ground, do not cross your hooked feet unless you can obtain a figure-four position (see illustration) and keep your legs on your opponent's thighs to prevent his applying ankle locks.

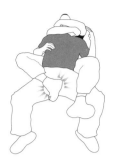

Rear-Mount Face Bar with Heel Kick to Groin

The face bar is a fearful attack from the rear mount targeting your opponent's face and neck.

From a rear mount you will pincer your legs around your opponent and clasp your forearms on the opponent's face just below his nose. Squeeze tightly and lean back, hyperextending his neck and placing extreme pressure on the jaw. Be sure to do this quickly and decisively because your forearms are exposed to his teeth.

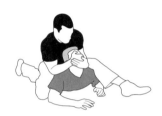

Neck Pressure from the Topside Rearmount

The neck pressure and crank is a move that may cause serious harm to your opponent's neck and spine.

Your opponent is on his stomach with you on top. Place your full weight on the opponent by straddling him with one leg and extending your other leg across the opponent's shoulder. You have the option of using an eye gouge or pressure to the philtrum with your middle fingers or cupping the hands to his chin to put extreme pressure on the neck. Note that straddling the opponent with only one leg allows you to torque his head backward and limits the ability of his back to arch, thereby putting more pressure on the neck. A two-legged straddle would make it more difficult to pull the opponent's head back using your upper-body weight shift and momentum backward. Do not apply pressure using an angle that would allow your opponent to counter by rolling over.

Counters to Defensive Measures Against Your Rear Naked Choke Attempt

If the opponent defends against your rear naked choke attempt by yanking down on your choking arm, you may use your other arm to exert a wrist lock to counter the defense.

If the opponent defends by yanking down on your choking arm, you may also grab your own clothing while repositioning your other arm underneath his chin to execute an opposite-arm choke. Basically, you are switching one choking arm for the other.

Defense Against an Opponent Attempting a Rearmount When You Are on All Fours

This defense is used when you are facedown on all fours and your opponent has his chest above your head while on top of you and is trying to mount you.

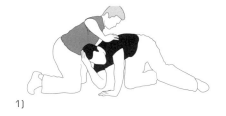

1)

From all fours, tuck your chin and drop onto your back by bringing one arm into your chest and spinning into a defensive position, positioning your knee and foreleg across the opponent's torso to keep him away from you. Continue with *retzev* counterattacks.

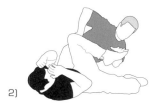

2)

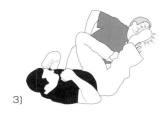

3)

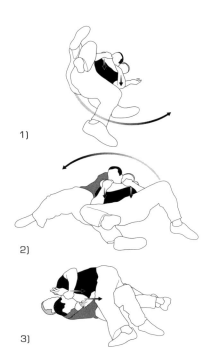

1)

2)

3)

Defense Against the Rear Mounted Naked Choke

When fighting on the ground, if an attacker takes your back, you are in grave danger of his applying a blood choke. A good ground fighter will pincer his legs around you to prevent your escape and extend his body by stretching his legs and upper body in opposite directions to strengthen the choke or face bar. You are also in jeopardy of the attacker delivering punishing heel kicks to your groin (as you might do to an opponent). A choke from the rear mount is one of the worst positions you can find yourself in, but it is not indefensible. However, it must be defended against immediately. Biting the attacker's forearm is a real and effective option to facilitate the release.

If you find yourself in this highly disadvantageous position, you must react immediately before the opponent can sink the choke and hook his legs around you to stretch your body out by extending his hips and leaning back with his upper body. Raise your right leg to prevent him from sinking his leg hooks into you. If he does sink his hooks, you must try to slide one of your legs inside a hooked foot and over it to break the hold. Repeat the same move with the other leg. Keep your chin tucked and yank down his choking arm with both of your arms prior to his sinking the choke. You may also rip a chunk out of his arm with your teeth. If he sinks the choke with his right arm, you must yank down on his right arm just above the wrist with your right arm and the biceps of his left arm. Continue to yank down on his right arm just above his elbow with your right arm and remove his left hand from the back of your head with your left hand. While defending against his initial choke attempt, you must bridge by raising your body on the balls of your feet and rolling into the crook of your attacker's elbow and onto your stomach to break the hold. You need to maneuver your body away from his choking elbow to create some space to turn back into the crook of his elbow, create separation, and defeat the choke. The turn onto your stomach must be forceful. The goal is to end up facing the

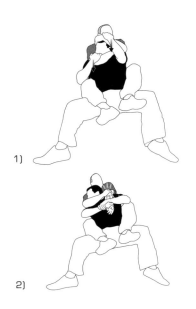

1)

2)

attacker, allowing counterattacks such as eye gouges, knee strikes, and other combatives. Once you create enough separation to comfortably breathe, counterattack his eyes and groin followed by *retzev.*

If your attacker is able to sink his leg hooks, a second option is to keep your chin tucked and use both arms to remove his left hand from the back of your head to counterattack with a straight arm bar over your shoulder. Again, bite his arm if the opportunity arises. Use your legs to push back and push your shoulders up to his torso to fight his grip. Note, you may also yank down on his hand, clutching his opposite bicep. Be sure to have defended against the choke adequately before going on the counteroffensive. Sliding your hips out will increase pressure on the arm. Be sure to keep his thumb pointed up. You must execute this move quickly because both of your hands are committed, leaving you vulnerable. While defending the choke, you may also slip your right leg around the opponent's right ankle and use your other leg for a strong figure four ankle lock.

Defense Against Being Drowned

Krav maga deals with worst-case assault scenarios. Being forcibly drowned is one of them. As with all assault situations, the best defense is to avoid the attack in the first place. *Krav maga* uses its principal choke defenses, with modifications, to counter chokes and drowning attempts. As in all ground fighting, at all costs you must prevent the opponent from taking your back. All of his weight may be used to force your head under water, especially if it is shallow water and he can mount you from the rear. You must turn your body to face the attacker while either plucking his hands away from your head and throat or clearing his hands by bringing your biceps to your ear while folding your forearm on top of your head and turning with all of your strength to get your face out of the water.

OFFENSIVE TECHNIQUES FROM THE MOUNT

When obtaining the mount, do not sit on your opponent. Keep your weight settled high on his chest to maintain balance and control his arms to help protect your groin with a forward lean. Your knees must provide good balance platforms as you hook your heels into the side of your opponent. In addition, your knees should be close to the opponent's torso and as high as possible toward the opponent's armpits to limit his striking and evasive abilities. (In defending against the mount, keep your elbows in to prevent the opponent from riding up the torso, as discussed later.) Place yourself in the best possible position to strike and control while defending your groin. Controlling the opponent's arms provides two tactical advantages: you can rain combative strikes down on his head and throat with impunity along with arm bar options and chokes, and you can prevent him from striking your groin. If you do not control your opponent's arms, you can still pierce his defenses to attack his head and throat. From the mount you have more mobility, and also gravity is on your side, allowing you to deliver withering combatives. It is highly advantageous to keep your opponent's back pinned to the ground to limit his escape options.

You can also position yourself with one knee on an opponent's arm while trapping his other arm to facilitate combatives. This option also allows for arm bar variations against the opponent's free arm, such as control hold to arm bar with a throat grab. For the arm bar throat grab technique on the ground, you will trap one of the opponent's arms with your knee or reverse the mount into a far-side arm bar.

The following points will help you to maintain and use the mount to your greatest advantage:

- To maintain the mount you must develop good balance to counter the opponent's body turns, hip bucks, and push releases. One of the most common defenses is for the opponent to buck or throw you using his hips to bridge. Note that this is a *krav maga* defense against a substandard mount.

- Another strong strategy is to keep the opponent's hands pinned forward and above his head with your upper body leaning into the opponent to protect your groin, but understand that your eyes, face, and throat are vulnerable to counterattack.

- If your weight is forward while you are using your arms as supports against the ground, your opponent may try to trap one of your arms to roll you to that same side. To counter this, you may "swim," or reposition your arms against his, performing a bridge and other escape attempts while keeping proper body posture, positioning, and balance. You can blade your body against push attempts by angling your torso to the side just as he is about to make contact with his hands.

- If your opponent tries to push you off him with both arms, you may deflect both of them using a variation of the L block parry punch defense (see page 49). This particular defense against the push renders your opponent highly vulnerable to an arm bar.

- If your weight is forward and your opponent attempts a low push, shift your weight forward and secure one of your arms around the opponent's neck.

- If your opponent attempts to push one of your straddling knees back, yank or pluck his hands up and away from your knees.

- If your opponent wishes to roll on his stomach, let him. Loosen your legs slightly to allow the opponent's movement; if you tighten them, he can throw or roll you over.

- If your opponent tries to close the distance between you by using a bear hug from the bottom, you can use eye gouges (similar to the standing defense) or apply a painful arm brace to the jaw and throat by bracing his face across the jaw with your forearm or using the heel of one or both palms. The same technique will work if the opponent tries to grab your neck; insert a brace to throat and jaw.

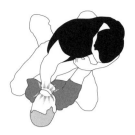

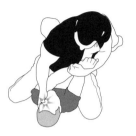

Trapping the Opponent's Arms for *Retzev* Combatives

Trapping the opponent's arms takes away his ability both to defend and to counterattack you, specifically your groin. You can deliver extreme punishment from this advantageous position.

Trap your opponent's arms by securing them firmly together against your body with the inside of your forearm. Strikes can include punches, palm heels, horizontal forearms, vertical elbows, and gouges to the head, neck, and eyes, along with arm-bar options. You can also execute groin strikes by turning your body and striking his exposed groin.

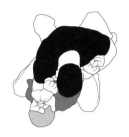

"GROUND AND POUND" DRILL

Straddle two large kicking pads and add a hand pad on top of both shields to simulate the head, or use a heavy bag laid on the ground. Use various combatives including straight punches, half-roundhouse punches, vertical elbows, hammer fists (using the fleshy underside of a clenched fist), and forearm strikes to simulate attacking your opponent. Practice pinning one of your arms to your chest to simulate trapping his arms. A partner may wish to help hold the shields in place along with the hand pad. This drill simulates both the mount and rear mount so that you can rain down strikes on an opponent.

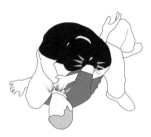

Brace to the Throat or Jaw

This powerful face bar puts extreme pressure against the throat or jaw.

This technique can be used to choke your opponent, attack his windpipe, or put strong pressure against his jaw. You will use your forearm against the opponent's throat or jaw by leaning forward, which protects your groin, and forcing the blade of the forearm into his throat for choking pressure. If the opponent tucks his chin, place the blade of your forearm against his near-side cheek and lean with all of your body weight into his jaw, creating an extremely painful face bar.

Defending Against the Brace to the Throat and Jaw

This simple but effective defense removes the pressure of the above described offensive technique.

Push the opponent's elbow across your face to alleviate the pressure on your jaw and throat. You have a reverse "baby pressure hold", which, if applied properly can choke your opponent from the bottom position. You can also roll into the top position for superior choking leverage.

Straight Arm Bars

Arm bars are one of the most highly effective and easy-to-execute ground combatives. Breaking pressure is effectively and easily applied.

From the mount, you can trap one or both of your opponent's arms while repositioning yourself to execute the arm bar. The following beginner straight arm bar variations trap the opponent's arm between your legs. Be sure the opponent's arm is positioned with his thumb up to best position his elbow for breaking pressure. You must keep the opponent's biceps and deltoid extremely close and tight to your hips before exerting pressure and leaning backward. Do not break contact between your inner thigh and the opponent's targeted arm. By pincering your legs around the arm and squeezing your knees together, you further isolate the joint while thwarting his ability to defend by turning in toward you or rolling to alleviate pressure on the arm. With less movement available from other connecting joints, the elbow becomes even more vulnerable. (The same isolation movement is true of other locks.) Breaking pressure is placed slightly above the opponent's elbow. When repositioning from the mount, keep pressure on the opponent's head with a thumb in the eye or cross face bar. Note that some arm bar variations place your lower leg in front of the opponent's face, providing him the opportunity to bite your leg—a definite *krav maga* option. Therefore, arm bars must be executed quickly and decisively, as is the case with all locks.

Here are a few armbar variations:

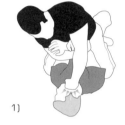

1)

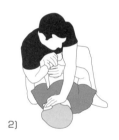

2)

1. **Basic.** Your opponent is flat on back and you have achieved a cross position by securing his targeted arm tightly between your legs. Keep your hips close to his body by positioning your thigh above his elbow. Squeeze your knees together to further isolate the joint's movement and push down on the ground with your heels. Clasp the opponent's arm tightly and lean back while simultaneously extending your hips up for breaking pressure.

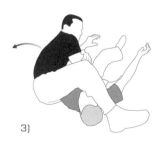

3)

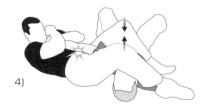

4)

2. **Scissors.** Crossing your legs can be used when your opponent is lying flat, trying to stand, or turning on his stomach. Locking your legs together provides powerful leg pincers, allowing you to extend your hips and torso together to exert breaking pressure.

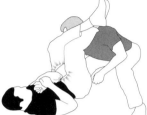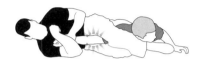

3. **L-brake.** After securing the opponent's arm, insert your far-side leg in front of his face, firmly pushing his head away with your shin. This also allows your free leg to deliver devastating heel kicks to the head.

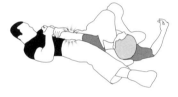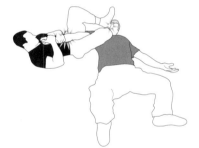

4. **Armbar feint.** From the mount you appear to focus on barring one arm and begin the initial movement of turning your body, but, switching directions and targeting the opposite arm will catch your opponent off-guard. As previously discussed, if the opponent pushes you with both of his arms, you are in a great position to execute an arm bar to either one or both of his extended arms from top mount position. You choose which arm is best for your attack. Slip your left leg over the opponent's face while pinning the targeted arm to your inner

thigh and pincer your right leg across his upper torso to secure the lock by squeezing your thighs together. If you were targeting your opponent's right arm, you would maneuver your left leg in front of his face and move to your left or the opponent's right. Keep your hips tight to the opponent's shoulder and squeeze your knees together.

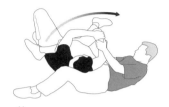

1)

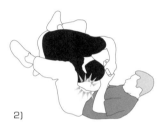

2)

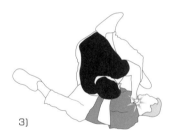

3)

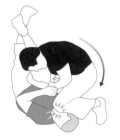

Variation when opponent still has the arm

Arm Bar Defenses

Basic Defense

The basic defense against the arm bar at the most elemental level is to prevent the opponent from grabbing and securing your arm. To defend against the straight arm bar technique variations, the instant you feel the opponent maneuvering for the arm bar, you must turn in toward your opponent with your elbow tip down, putting pressure directly into the opponent's groin. Simultaneously reach through his legs with your other arm, clasping your hands to ensure that your elbow is protected. You must not allow your opponent to pincer his legs because he will have other strong options available from this position. If the arm bar is executed properly by pincering the legs, all of his weight and core strength will be concentrated on destroying your elbow.

Stacking Defense

A second defense is used if you find yourself in a kneeling or standing position in the opponent's guard with your arm caught between the attacker's legs. You will use a compression technique against your opponent's spine to force all of your weight forward, preventing the attacker from extending his hips while protecting your arm by breaking the angle of attack, keeping your arm bent, and clasping it tight to your body with your other free arm. Jam the tip of your elbow into his throat. You must keep turning into the opponent to place him in the most precarious and contorted position possible. The technique puts tremendous pressure on his neck and spine. This combined weight forward and pressure will give you the opportunity to maneuver your body slightly to the side and launch combatives such as knees to the tailbone and lower back or stomps to the attacker's head. (Your opponent can also maneuver to keep pressure on the arm, and remove pressure from his neck, so beware.)

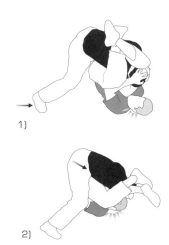

A third defense if the attacker succeeds in hooking his elbow inside your elbow while pincering his legs around your arm is to clasp both of your arms tight at the elbows. This is tricky because there are many counters to this defense, including wrist locks to release your defensive grip or your opponent using one of his legs to kick through one of your arms, forcing you to release. In any event, this purely defensive position is difficult to maintain for any length of time. It is best used as a stopgap measure—you must react quickly as the opponent countermaneuvers. Lastly, you may execute a backward roll over the shoulder of your trapped arm if the opponent has one leg draped over your head; however, you must do this decisively because your opponent can easily reposition himself to continue the attack.

The fundamental principle supporting joint locks is to use one's entire mass and strength against the opponent's joint. Do not let this happen to you. To be sure, strength will help in both attacking and defending, but technique is the only sure way to win. Note also that there are numerous countertechniques to these basic defenses.

DEFENSES AGAINST THE MOUNT

Defenses against the mount and sidestraddle knee on stomach (where the opponent has his knee on your midsection with all of his weight on you) are critical. You must think of your "fighting chess game" and how your opponent will look for a dominant position. Accordingly, you must use techniques to avoid being mounted and side-straddled, and especially having your arms trapped.

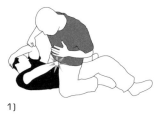

1)

Mount Defense Strikes to the Groin

Attack your opponent's groin immediately with punches and downward elbow strikes.

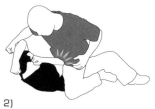

2)

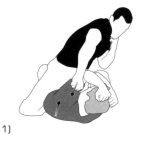

1)

Cover Your Head with Forearms, Defend and Deflect with Body Movement, and Counterstrike

While similar to upper-body defenses, defending strikes from the mount requires you to shift your body weight to avoid being a stationary target. Never keep your back flat to the ground; always remain slightly raised and on your side to ensure the possibility of movement. You must counterstrike immediately and attempt to bridge by raising your hips to one side with the help of your shoulder, facing the direction in which you hope to launch your opponent. This can be challenging if your opponent carries

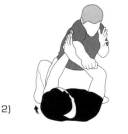

2)

a considerable weight and strength advantage. Cover your head with your forearms, keeping your elbows in to defend against strikes and arm bars, while using body movement by shifting side to side and snaking with hip buck to dismount or unbalance the attacker. This technique also sets up a vertical elbow to the opponent's groin and prevents the opponent from gaining the high mount.

Bear-Hug Opponent and Turnover Pin for Counterattacks

Pinning one of the opponent's arms and squeezing your bodies together, roll the opponent over on his side, and follow with additional combatives. A knee combative to the groin and coccyx will also help roll your opponent.

You must close the distance with your opponent by clinching him tightly. Think of your opponent as a table with four supports: two knees and two arms. If you remove one of his arm supports, he is vulnerable to being turned in that direction. Roll him and continue with counterattacks, including additional knee and hand groin strikes, leg locks, and other combatives.

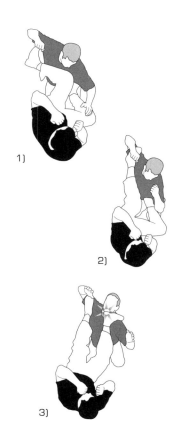

1)

2)

3)

> *Note: More advanced techniques will provide the defender with counterstrikes and arm bars; however, the attacker can also use counters such as wedging his heels and shifting his body weight to avoid being dislodged.*
>
> *Never* turn facedown and expose the back of your neck to an attacker.

Use Horizontal Knee Brace to Disengage and Create Distance

The "brakes" technique disengages you from an attacker who is trying to mount you or spread your legs.

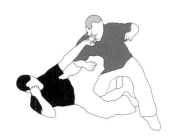

Turn on your side and raise one leg to use your shin and knee to keep an attacker at bay as you deliver combatives such as eye gouges, throat strikes, punches, knee strikes, and kicks. This is a strong defense, because you can use all four of your limbs to defend. Your hips and legs are your most powerful muscle groups. As you separate yourself from your attacker, forcefully extend your shin and patella to both strike and push away from your opponent. You will likely gain the opportunity to kick him in the groin or head using your underneath leg or in the head using a straight kick with the heel or a modified side kick while on the ground, again using the heel. Make contact with the groin, midsection or face. Get up immediately by sliding your underneath leg back and onto the ball of your foot while posting one hand on the ground and keeping one hand up to deliver more combatives and make your escape.

FROM THE GUARD

Defense Against Roundhouse Punch into Control Hold 2 from the Guard

This highly effective technique defends against an opponent who has the mount and is throwing a roundhouse punch at your head.

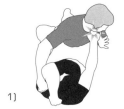

1)

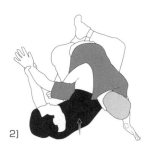

2)

Use an outside forearm block with your left arm against a right roundhouse punch while simultaneously delivering counterpunches to the opponent's head or groin. With your opponent held in the closed guard, you may time the punch and use your pincered legs to pull your opponent off balance into you with this technique. This technique sets up a prone variation of Control Hold 2 (page 103) by securing his arm while clamping down on his shoulder and releasing the closed guard momentarily to turn on your side and gain maximum positional control, then reclosing the guard.

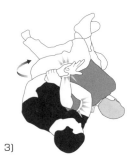

3)

COMBINING TECHNIQUES: THE CAVALIER INTO STRAIGHT ARM BAR

Try combining the cavalier takedown with an arm bar follow-up using extreme control and caution. After the opponent is down, immediately insert your far-side leg around his target arm. Enormous breaking pressure will come from your controlled fall by applying maximum breaking force to your opponent's elbow fulcrum while tightly wedged against your inner thigh. Be sure to keep your hips close to his armpit. When practicing with a partner do not at any time keep the partner's arm straight. Even the slightest pressure can seriously damage your partner's elbow with this combination.

THE *KRAV MAGA* CLOSED HIGH GUARD

Krav maga recognizes that you may end up on your back in a fight. So you must be capable of defending against all manners of combatives, especially strikes and chokes. When you close your guard by wrapping one ankle around the other, if you react quickly to protect your groin by pulling your opponent's torso close to you, the guard position offers many offensive capabilities, including upper-body strikes and heel kicks to your opponent's kidneys. Perhaps two of the most effective locks when trapping one or both of your opponent's arms from the closed guard are immediate transition to the arm bar and triangular choke variations. Controlling your attacker with your legs pincered high around his torso can have great tactical advantages.

You must maneuver quickly, because when defending against an opponent using the guard we strike to the groin immediately. You must not allow this to happen to you. Immediately transition to the offense and close the distance to prevent strikes to your vulnerable areas, or ride your opponent to prevent him from getting a shot at your groin. The closed-guard pincer can help level the fighting field when facing a powerful and heavy opponent. There are myriad possible offenses from the closed guard. We will focus on a few core techniques and their corresponding counter-defenses.

Arm Bar Transition by Sliding Legs up and Across the Face from the High Closed Guard

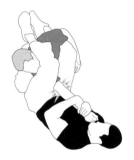

An upright arm bar variation using the right arm as the example may be executed by swinging your left leg over (right leg for the left arm bar) and isolating the attacker's right arm by wrapping your leg around his left shoulder (right shoulder for the left arm-bar) and crossing your other leg at the ankles to pincer the arm. This brings your body perpendicular to your opponent's, setting up the optimal arm bar angle. Once the arm is securely pincered, extend your hips and clamp down with your hamstrings and heels, driving down to apply breaking pressure to the arm. A variation of this technique involves taking the leg on the same side as the attacker's arm and hooking your shin and ankle under the attacker's chin while thrusting your leg into his throat or jaw to exert breaking pressure.

Neck Crank from the High Closed Guard

The neck crank from the guard can have serious consequences for your opponent, especially if you keep your legs pincered.

While on your back, you have drawn your opponent into facing you between your pincered legs. Securing your opponent's head from its rear into your chest, you will force your opponent's chin sideways while your other arm reaches around to secure his forehead or near-side eye socket. Torque or crank his neck forcefully to the side.

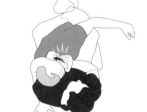

1)

Note: This powerful technique is also readily available from the inside clinch.

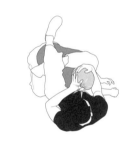

2)

Triangular Leg Choke with Combatives

Triangular leg chokes are an extremely powerful combative, utilizing your strongest muscle groups and core strength against an opponent's vulnerable neck.

You can use the triangular leg choke, one of the most formidable offensive techniques, when you are on your back, your opponent is between your legs, and you control one of his arms. Your legs and hips can exert unparalleled choking pressure on the trapped opponent's neck. Upper-body combatives can also be added. Because this technique requires some hip flexibility, it is particularly well suited for women. Keeping the opponent's arm trapped between your legs is fundamental because the opponent's own shoulder will be instrumental in applying the choking pressure.

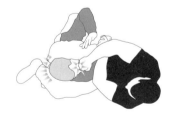

Your left leg (the same side as the opponent's extended shoulder) will extend straight out and pin his right shoulder. Your other leg will loop over the opponent's other shoulder and wrap around the back of his neck to touch the back of the knee of your extended leg. Close your extended leg down on the ankle of your

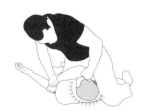

looped leg, forming a leg vise or figure four. You can use your same-side hand to pull your leg through at the shin to help exert pressure. Maneuver your body slightly to the side of your looped-over leg, which will create a better angle for the choke. Clamp down hard, forcing your knees and thighs together. Similar to the neck clinch, place both hands on the top of the opponent's skull and pull his head into your midsection.

If your opponent tries to stand up to defend against the triangle, bridge your body by extending your hips to continue the choke. You may also release one of your arms to yank his Achilles tendon to put him on his back. Should you perform this technique, you must move with him. If you must take him back down in this manner, do not lose the choke or disengage. The triangular leg choke can also be applied with an opponent on his side as you turn with him. You should also launch combative strikes, including punches and eye gouges to the opponent's head to better exert the choke.

If you lose the triangular choke because of your opponent's counterpositioning or make the tactical decision to disengage while maintaining control of the arm, transitioning to an arm bar is readily available by crossing your same-side leg across the opponent's face to pincer your legs. You may also apply a triangular choke from the mount by inserting one leg behind your opponent's neck while trapping his arm and hooking the other leg over the top of the crossed leg.

Basic Release Against Triangular Leg Choke

Once again, you must not allow anyone to get his hand, arms, or legs around your neck. If it happens, you must disengage through leverage.

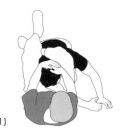

1)

The best defense against a triangle leg choke is to avoid being placed in one in the first place. Nevertheless, if you find yourself in this dangerous position, you must attack your opponent's eyes immediately with your free hand and try to create separation with your trapped arm if you can manage it. You can also stand to compress your attacker's neck, but he can move as well to counter this defense (as we would in our defense against this technique). Attacking the opponent's eyes, while highly effective, does not guarantee success because the opponent can block your attacks as well (as you would for an opponent trying to attack your eyes). Another defense requiring power and leverage is to lift your opponent as soon as he attempts the hold and slam his head and neck hard into the ground. A word to the wise: do not get caught in this hold.

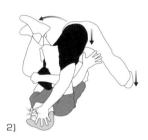

2)

Front Ground Headlock Choke or "Guillotine" from the High Guard

The front ground headlock with leg pincers, otherwise known as the "guillotine," is a dominant position from which to choke an opponent. You may also deliver debilitating heel kicks to an opponent's kidneys.

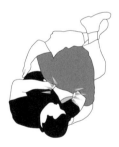

You are on your back with your opponent facing you between your legs with a high guard pincering your legs around his upper torso. Your right arm is encircling the opponent's neck with the blade of your forearm across the opponent's throat beneath his chin. Exert choking pressure on his windpipe using the blade of your forearm by keeping the choking arm's thumb pointed up. The other arm is pulled tight with your opposite hand clasping your encircling arm's wrist. Forcefully pull your right arm up and

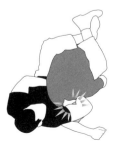

Variation

into your chest. Your left shoulder is slightly off the ground as you exert pressure on the opponent's neck. Your back is not flat against the ground due to your shoulder upturn and hip placement. Pincer your legs to better pull him in toward you and secure him while extending his body to facilitate the choke. Lean back to squeeze the choke by pulling his head in with your choking arm and lifting your other elbow up. You also have the option of heel attacks to your opponent's kidneys.

Note: This choke may also be executed with your non-choking arm under the opponent's armpit.

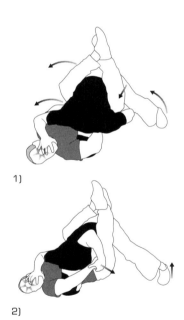

1)

2)

Release Against Front Ground Headlock or "Guillotine" Choke

The best way to counter this attack—as with all attacks—is not to be put into it. As noted, this is an extremely dangerous position for you. However, there are some defensive options.

The initial defensive release against the front headlock with choke is to immediately break the angle of attack with your body, preventing your opponent from pincering his legs. Turn your head into the crook of his elbow to allow yourself more breathing space. Use your arm closest to his choking arm to yank his arm down to relieve the pressure on your throat while simultaneously using your top-side arm to attack his eyes. You may also deliver a right knee strike to his tailbone. Try to drive the shoulder of your arm attacking your opponent's face into him to help break the choke. If possible, rising on the balls of your feet will help counter his pressure against your throat and provide additional force into his eye socket. Finish with *retzev* strikes and other combatives, including counters with your own joint break locks.

Variation: You are caught in the front ground headlock. Defend by creating a face bar with the opposite arm to the attacker's choking forearm (if he is choking with his left arm, your will defend with your right and attack his face with your left) while simultaneously yanking down on the guillotining arm and keeping your elbow firmly pressed into the attacker's thigh to alleviate pressure. Knee the attacker repeatedly in the groin or coccyx. Finish with retzev *strikes and other combatives, including your own joint break locks.*

Variation: If the attacker succeeds in pinning one of your arms inside his legs, you must continue to turn onto your side and yank down on the attacker's arm with your free arm to alleviate pressure. Continue to fight your way out but do not turn onto your back. This is definitely a difficult hold to defend.

DEFENSES AGAINST THE OPPONENT'S CLOSED GUARD

Groin Strikes in the Closed Guard

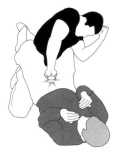

If you maintain proper upright body position, the opponent's groin is open to strikes.

"Posture up" by seating your weight back and remaining upright to rudely jam your knee into your opponent's tail bone. This can be a debilitating strike in itself and a counter against your opponent's attempt to control you with his legs. Strike your opponent's groin using straight punches, hammer fists, and vertical elbows along with grabs and twists. You may also trap one or both of the opponent's arms while delivering simultaneous combatives. Note again, these combatives set up powerful leglock techniques. The high closed guard can allow your opponent strong body control over you, placing you in a highly vulnerable position.

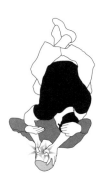

Eye Gouges if Opponent Pulls You into His Closed Guard

If your opponent successfully breaks your posture and clinches your head, use thumb gouges to the eyes to disengage, followed by *retzev* including an immediate strike to the throat.

Note: The same eye gouge technique can be used if someone grabs you around the waist with your arms free, except you shoot back your hips or, alternatively, hook one leg around the attacker and blade your body to the side to create a stronger base.

LEG AND ANKLE LOCKS

Leglocks, if skillfully and forcefully applied to the ankle and knee, can sever tendons and ligaments. However, controlling the legs' powerful muscles is generally more difficult and requires more power than arm locks. The principles involved in locking the knee and ankle are similar to those underlying wrist and arm locks. Attacking the ankle can cause separation of muscle and tendons. Dislocating the knee damages the four main ligaments and misaligns the bones. Boots can complicate ankle locks, but if the lock is applied properly, it can still be executed while placing additional torque on the knee. Similar to the elbows, the knees are the leg's vulnerable spot. Lateral pressure is optimally applied to cause the most damage. In practice, you must work carefully with your partner because the pain from leg and ankle locks takes longer to register and you can injure your partner by the time he feels significant pain.

Rear Leg Lock Folding Opponent's Legs with Weight Against Them and Choke

You can also combine leg locks with chokes to further negate your opponent's ability to defend and counterattack.

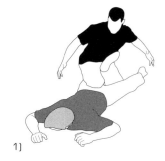

1)

The facedown knee lock involves inserting your own leg as an impediment while forcing the opponent's knee forward against the knee's full natural movement. Insert your outside leg into the crook of the opponent's bent knee and wrap your inserted leg's ankle behind your opponent's leg. By leaning forward you will put tremendous pressure on the opponent's knee while placing yourself in position to execute a choke or neck crank variation. You may also cross both of your opponent's legs and exert pressure forward.

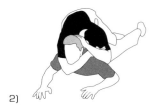

2)

Achilles Leg Bar

This bar targets the Achilles tendon and can often be applied as a surprise counterattack.

The Achilles leg bar is an effective counterattack against an opponent who has tried to pull you into his guard or has gone to ground with you. It can be applied as a surprise attack as soon as you go to ground with your attacker. Encircle and trap the opponent's leg with your arm and place the blade of your forearm just above the opponent's ankle, digging it into his Achilles tendon. Be sure to place the bony radial part of your wrist directly behind and slightly above the ankle, targeting the Achilles tendon. There are several grip options to secure the opponent's leg. I prefer grabbing my free arm with my engaged arm while placing my non-gripping hand against the opponent's shin and placing my foot into his crotch with a heel kick. You must not allow any separation or space between your encirclement and his leg. Squeeze the targeted leg tightly with both arms to apply significant pressure to the Achilles tendon. Pincer your legs around your opponent's

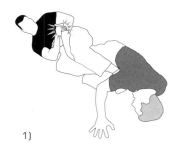

1)

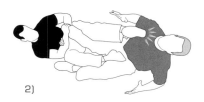

2)

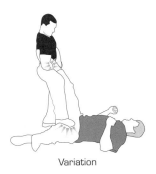

Variation

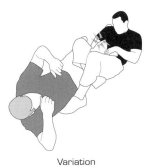

Variation

targeted leg, resting them on his opposite lower thigh to make the lock harder to defend against.

If flexibility allows, a high pincer movement with your same-side leg will make it harder to defend against the lock by making it more difficult for the opponent to unwrap your legs. After your grip is secure, you will lean back. This body torque, if applied quickly and violently, will rupture or sever the tendon. It is best to turn the opponent on his side to trap his free leg and prevent him from kicking you in an effort to escape.

The Achilles leg bar may also be executed while an opponent is on the ground and you are standing. In this case, you want to execute the bar against his leg while to his outside. Do not attempt the bar while straddling his free leg because he can kick you in the groin. You can also apply the bar to an opponent who is standing over you while you are on the ground by cinching the Achilles tendon tightly and using your legs to unbalance or take down your opponent.

Defense Against Achilles Leg Bar

To prevent your opponent from securing the Achilles leg bar, the moment you feel his attempt, kick hard to loosen his grip while simultaneously preventing him from pincering his legs. At the same time use combatives, including kicking your opponent in the head with your free leg. As you kick through to disengage from the lock attempt, you may want to kneel up into the attacker to finish with *retzev* combatives, including a diagonally placed knee strike and upper-body combatives to the opponent's head along with arm bar options. You can also apply an ankle lock to his far-side leg, as described next.

If you are standing and your opponent is on the ground kicking at you, you can secure a standing-falling lock by cinching the lock and then falling to the ground, creating tremendous pressure on the Achilles tendon. As noted, you must stand to the oppo-

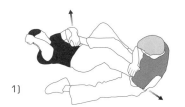

1)

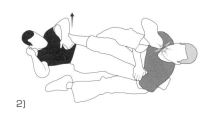

2)

nent's side when trapping his leg to prevent being kicked in the groin; do not stand so that his other leg is between your legs. The falling Achilles lock will sever the Achilles tendon because of the tremendous pressure exerted by the fall.

A defense against a standing-falling lock where your opponent has your leg and is preparing to drop to the ground to increase the pressure is to grab the opponent's near leg and execute your own preemptive lock immediately by tightening around the opponent's Achilles tendon and leaning back to preempt the lock.

Ankle-Heel Lock

Ankle and heel locks are also a highly effective combative to dislocate the ankle and rupture tendons and ligaments.

Ankle-heel locks, sometimes known as "toe holds," are often preceded by a takedown and are a highly effective default lock when an Achilles lock attempt fails. The heel hook is a highly effective technique attacking the ligaments of the knee in addition to the ankle. Trap the opponent's toe in your armpit while snaking one arm underneath and around his heel. Clasp your other arm and draw the ankle tightly into your body while torquing to the inside. This ankle-heel lock will place tremendous pressure on the knee ligaments.

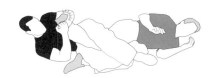

Note: The inside heel hook is easily transitioned to from the Achilles leg bar. You will simply release the intended Achilles bar and encircle your arm around the ankle to exert breaking pressure.

OFFENSES FROM THE SIDE MOUNT

Knee Combatives Chest Down

These devastating combatives can be delivered to an opponent while he is on his back with his midsection exposed while you are pressing him to the ground with your chest down.

Chest down atop your opponent, you have a strong stable platform from which to attack your opponent's groin, midsection, eyes, and head with knees, elbows, gouges, and fists along with joint attacks and chokes while also protecting your groin. For a side mount to your opponent's right, keep your right knee pressed to your opponent's hip. Your left knee is in line with your opponent's head (ideal for modified roundhouse knee strikes). Your same-side elbow should be positioned on your opponent's ear (ideal for vertical drop elbow combatives) along with punches and attacking your opponent's eyes. The side mount also nicely sets up the mount.

Defenses against the sidemount include knees to your opponent's midsection and eye attacks. A triangular leg choke may also be available if you succeed in forcing your opponent's head away from you into the crook of your knee.

It is important to position yourself on the ball of your grounded foot to add power and extension to the strike. To defend against these devastating knee strikes if momentarily caught in this position, bring your near-side knee to your chest to create a brace, blocking the incoming knee with your shin. Do not stay in this position, however.

Baby Pressure Triangular Choke and Cervical Pressure Holds from the Side Mount

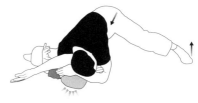

1)

This blood choke/pressure hold exerts choking and crushing vertebral pressure when the opponent's arm is either trapped or free.

This technique puts you in a dominant position by securing the opponent's near-side arm and driving your shoulder through this arm to apply strangulation pressure against the neck. Similar to the guillotine lock, your right arm is clasping the left arm. You will drive your shoulder into your opponent's chin while propping yourself on the balls of both feet to increase the strangulation pressure on his neck. Damaging knee strikes to the opponent's midsection can be added. As noted above, bury your head to protect your eyes.

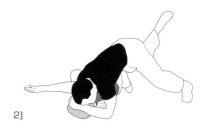

2)

A variation of this technique is applied when your opponent is on his back and you are to his side with your right forearm around his neck with the blade of your right forearm pressed at the base of his skull. Your left arm is clasping the right arm. You will drive your shoulder into his chin while propping yourself on the balls of both feet to increase the inward pressure on his neck.

Damaging knee strikes can once again be applied to the opponent's midsection. Bury your head to protect your eyes.

Note: Both of these variations can be done from the mount.

OTHER MOVES

Knee on the Stomach with Combatives Trapping Opponent's Arm

The knee on the stomach is a highly effective position to deliver punishing combatives to the opponent's head, throat, and groin.

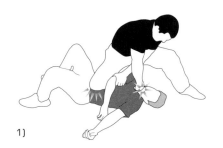

1)

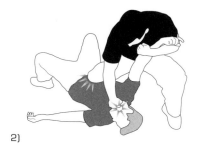

2)

By placing your full weight onto your opponent's midsection and hooking your foot into your opponent's hip, you create a stable striking platform and wear down your opponent's body by digging your weight into his midsection. Your other leg is positioned diagonally to your opponent's leg and bent at approximately a 45-degree angle providing a strong base. Optimally, you should pin his arm closest to you to protect your groin. (As a defense against this position, you should not allow your near-side arm to be trapped so you can attack the opponent's groin.) Another option is to trap the opponent's arm on your thigh to deliver withering combatives, providing the option of sinking a straight arm bar.

The Ground Side Headlock
with Combatives

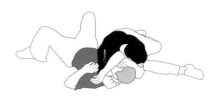

The ground side headlock establishes a good base by exerting tremendous pressure on an opponent's cervical vertebrae while also setting up an opponent for retzev *ground combatives.*

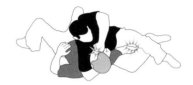

Variation

Encircle your right arm around the opponent's neck splaying your right (underneath) leg out with the knee bent close to your opponent's head and the outside of your foot touching the ground. Your left leg is splayed wide while keeping the inside foot touching the ground, giving you a strong base of operation. Both of your knees are bent 90 degrees. Keep your head close to avoid countertechniques such as eye gouges and anything else you might try if you were in your opponent's position. Take your right (underside) leg and hook it over your opponent's inside arm. Once the hook is complete, overlap your left leg and clamp down, placing breaking pressure on the arm and shoulder joint. Another option is to overhook your opponent's arm with your left leg to deliver punches with the option of a straight arm bar by squeezing your knees together. You can release control of the arm to deliver debilitating knee strikes to the head.

Release Against Side Ground Headlock

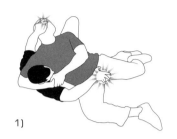

1)

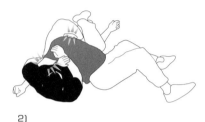

2)

Always keeping the fighting chess game in mind, krav maga *has countertechniques to the groundwork we teach. The best release against this attack—like every other attack—is not to be put into it. Remember one of the most important rules of self-defense: whatever you can do to someone, he can use to harm you.*

The defense against the side ground requires you to tuck your chin to protect your neck while simultaneously striking the opponent's groin and reaching around to attack the opponent's eyes or philtrum. Do not push against his chin; he will have power to resist using his neck muscles. A powerful follow-up is a modified triangular choke by raising your outside leg and hooking his throat in the crook of your knee while securing his other arm for an arm bar break. You may also deliver *retzev* strikes.

Note: As a countermeasure to defend against the ground headlock, do not allow your arm to be hooked. Another countermeasure is to preempt the opponent's obtaining the lock by forcing the opponent's head between your legs so you can apply a neck lock with your legs.

Release Against Side Ground Headlock with Arms Pinned

There is also a variation against the side ground headlock if your opponent has your arm pinned. You must maneuver your body to catch the opponent's legs. Once you have caught the legs, you will turn in toward your opponent while placing your outside arm across his face to execute an eye gouge or face bar to release his hold and put you in a position for *retzev* counterattacks. You can also deliver simultaneous knees to the opponent's kidneys. You may also trap the arm and then lean back into a straight arm bar.

A second variation is to pivot your body away from your opponent's torso (in this case, counterclockwise) and fishhook his eyes with both of your hands to yank his head back, forcing him to release you.

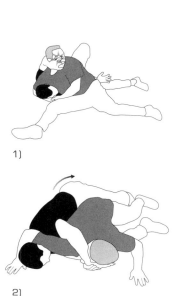

1)

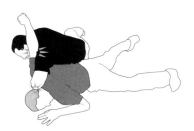

2)

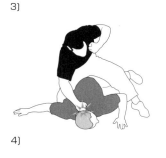

3)

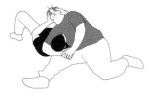

4)

5)

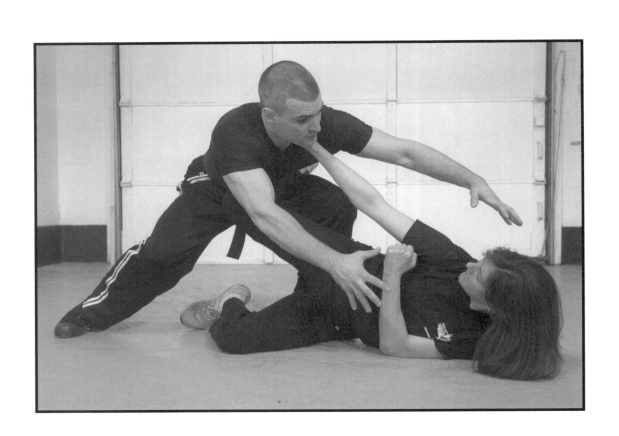

CHAPTER 8

Women's Self-Defense Principles

The force is with you—and someone else is feeling it.

While this chapter examines *krav maga* techniques and strategies specifically tailored for women, the techniques are applicable for everyone. Also, keep in mind that all the techniques from the previous chapters are every bit as effective for women as men. This chapter examines a few of the most common self-defense situations against unarmed attacks.

Violence against women often involves close proximity or infighting, especially during a sexual assault. While *krav maga* teaches the same techniques to both men and women, infighting and specialized ground techniques are particularly emphasized. Once again, mind-set is the key. With a strong mind and attitude you can protect your body and not give in to a victim mentality. You'll become the proverbial "hard target" rather than a "soft target." At all times exercise your intuition, good judgment, and common sense. Your safety is a primordial concern that will trigger your defensive actions. The intensity of your response will escalate to meet the threat.

Empower Your Mind; Protect Your Body™

Being proactive overcomes victimization. If you perceive a potential threat, take action and extricate yourself. The best defense against any attack is avoiding or removing yourself from the precarious situation. Only environmental awareness can help you do that. In an unfamiliar environment, check for threats, paying particular attention to potential adversaries' proximity and hand movements. Make use of your peripheral vision and constantly assess your surroundings.

In a potentially dangerous situation, quickly observe and assess. For example, is a weapon present? Is an escape route immediately available? Is the assailant intoxicated or under the influence of drugs? Is the assailant angry or bizarrely calm? What demands are being made? Are you confident of your ability to physically resist? The techniques in this book will begin to give you the skills and confidence to defend yourself.

A surprise attack will force you to react from an unprepared state. Therefore, your self-defense reaction must come from instincts and reflexes. *Krav maga* training prepares you for just that. The most important lesson *krav maga* can teach you is to not be taken by surprise in the first place. Becoming an accomplished observer helps you resolve a situation before it gets out of hand. By constantly surveying your locale, you'll be aware at all times of who and what surrounds you. Know that empathizing with or issuing an emotional appeal to an attacker carries considerable risk: an emotional appeal can spur on an attack rather than thwart it. Keep in mind that many female victims know their attackers. Also, sexual predators and other attackers often approach their victims with innocuous behavior such as friendly conversation.

Ignoring unsolicited entreaties will serve you well. You need not be civil if your instincts tell you to behave otherwise. Assertiveness is essential and one of the most effective strategies for preventing assault. If you lack assertiveness, you can develop it by working on your body posture. Holding your head high, presenting a comfortable and confident demeanor, maintaining eye contact, and moving with a confident stride makes it less likely that an attacker will see you as a potential victim. Learning *krav maga* is one sure way to build your confidence, assertiveness, and ability to withstand a physical assault. Most important, *krav maga* develops a paramount fighting attitude.

If you look your would-be attacker in the eyes and your body language conveys the message "I will not be a victim," you'll meet the potential threat head-on. (Strategically, however, such confrontational behavior runs the risk of escalating a situation.) Equally important, an assailant generally does not expect you to unleash *retzev* or a continuous, seamless, integrated, and concerted counterattack to stop him.

Twenty Commonsense Suggestions to Minimize Your Risk of Attack

1. If you are uncomfortable in a situation, leave. Use all of your senses to identify threats.
2. If someone is too close, create distance between yourself and the person. Keep your hands free.
3. Do not enter an elevator or closed environment with anyone who makes you uncomfortable.
4. If someone is following you, move to a heavily trafficked public place.
5. Avoid traveling alone at night or taking an unknown shortcut through a less densely populated area.
6. Be particularly vigilant in public restrooms, especially those with free access.
7. Avoid allowing anyone wishing to sell something to approach you.
8. Do not provide any information to strangers, especially personal information.
9. Should a vehicle approach, especially if the door is open, stay away.
10. In a parking lot, walk against the directional arrows to keep cars moving toward you. Keep your keys in your hand, and park your car facing out for rapid departure.
11. If someone attempts to grab you, scream and attract as much attention as possible.
12. When carrying a bag, place the shoulder strap across your chest. Try not to display money or expensive items in public.
13. Do not wear earphones in an unfamiliar environment.
14. If you are lost, approach a public official or enter a store to ask for directions.
15. In a risky situation, it is always a good idea to have an open phone line so that someone can summon help or call 911. However, do not engage in a conversation beyond alerting the person that you are in a potentially precarious situation.
16. Note that alcohol and violence often go together. You should be aware of closing time for bars to avoid placing yourself in harm's way.
17. Lock your doors and windows, both in your vehicle and at home.

18.   Require visitors to identify themselves.
19.   Fight with the determination that your life is at stake.
20.   Above all, trust your instincts.

While you need not live in fear, denial is the most common obstacle to taking appropriate action, which is why you must be prepared to face a violent situation. You must sharpen your mental and physical skills until you can call on them without thinking. With practice, when necessary you'll be able to explode into action. Your opponent will not know what hit him—repeatedly. Only serious, hard, and appropriate training can trigger this fighting response.

If *krav maga* is necessary, you must summon the courage and determination to fight for your life. If someone threatens you, especially with a weapon, you must make a decision: comply, escape, or fight. Weapon defenses are an integral part of the *krav maga* system but not the focus of this book. If you must fight, you must identify the opportune moment to attack—and continue attacking. Exert maximum speed and aggression. Your goal is not to definitively win a fight but to escape.

Krav maga hones your mental and physical skills. With correct training, you'll learn to conquer your fear to control the energy and power from your body's fight-or-flight response. You will learn not to freeze under pressure. When in danger, your brain and body respond reflexively. If you are in a fight and an opponent makes an unanticipated or unrecognized action, the brain cannot find a practiced response, resulting in decision paralysis. By training to respond, you will be able to call upon your reflexes when attacked. It is unusual to be in a situation where you have to fight for your life, but it does happen, and it certainly pays to be prepared.

You must personalize the *krav maga* techniques and make them your own. Choose the ballistic strikes and other combatives you

TRUE KRAVIST

IKMA instructor Katherina Guttman responds to a few questions. Kat is the first woman to complete the international instructor course in Israel under Grandmaster Haim Gidon.

What motivated you to learn krav maga?

As a fitness specialist, I continually seek various ways to challenge my fitness level; as an independent woman, I am intrigued by activities that develop self-empowerment. *Krav maga* is the official fighting system of the Israeli army and it offers a full body workout like no other. On discovering *krav maga,* I found a way to fulfill both my fitness and empowerment needs.

How important is it for women to learn self-defense? Is it enough just to take sensible and safe precautions?

It is not only important but essential for a woman to know how to defend herself. It is unfortunate that we live in a world where vigilance is necessary. It is helpful to learn how to avoid a dangerous situation with awareness training, but it is not enough. A woman must know how to protect herself in any situation.

In what way does krav maga offer a more comprehensive approach to the subject of female self-protection?

Krav maga is a system like no other because it was developed to easily teach self-defense skills to every member of the population—men, women, and children alike. Since *krav maga* focuses on technique rather than strength, women find it extremely easy to learn. Women learn everything men do, with additional sexual assault defenses. After just a few hours, a woman will be proficient in elbows, knees, kicks, and various strikes. She will also be able to defend against many basic attacks, including chokes, grabs, and assaults. She will be able to put her attacker down using *retzev,* an overwhelming continuous counterattack. It is not enough to know two techniques. One must be able to react to a myriad of attacks. One must also know enough to take out an attacker.

Many women don't believe that any self-defense system, including krav maga, *will prevail if they are attacked by a large, physically stronger, and aggressive male. What are your personal feelings and thoughts on this?*

Again, *krav maga* differs from any other system in that it was designed for every segment of the population, regardless of gender, size, and strength. Not only have I heard personal stories from women who were trained in *krav maga* and used it for protection, I have personal experience to confirm its validity. I spent three weeks in Israel in July 2005 training and fighting with men who are much stronger, taller, and heavier than I am. I was the only female amongst seventeen men to go through the international instructor's course given by Grandmaster Haim Gidon. I was honored to spend days learning and practicing the techniques under the training of Grandmaster Gidon and his top instructors. I must admit that I thought I had a great deal to prove upon my arrival. Being the only female amongst seventeen men, I had to prove that I could hold my own. I often had to be stronger, tougher, and more aggressive than the others to gain respect from the testosterone-saturated room. I punched, kicked, and grappled with men almost twice my size. When I found myself mounting a six-foot-five, 235-pound man after throwing him to the ground to pound him, I felt a sense of strength that can come only from inner confidence and mastered technique. By the end of the course we were all convinced that these techniques were more valuable than any weight, height, or strength advantage.

We seem to focus on the subject of rape, yet this isn't the only type of assault/intimidation (physical and verbal) that women face. Could you give us some examples of how krav maga *deals with other types of threats/assaults women face?*

When one addresses the issue of assaults against women, one usually focuses on the horrors and dangers of sexual assault. While rape continues to be a foremost issue, women face a plethora of attacks and violations, both physical and verbal. Stealing one's purse, groping, swearing, and insulting are all attacks that confront women. *Krav maga* offers defenses against these and many other female-specific attacks.

Continued on next page

Are women more acutely aware of the potential for violence in situations and environments? Can such situational awareness lead to their having the feeling of being a "victim in waiting"? If so, what solutions to this can krav maga *offer?*

I strongly believe that 95 percent of a woman's defense is self-confidence. I often describe this scene to my students and clients: An assailant who is searching for a victim may see five potential victims in his area. If four of them are walking with their head up high, exuding self-confidence, and the fifth one is walking with his or her head down, with a shy demeanor, this individual will be targeted by the assailant. One of the most valuable things *krav maga* provides is a greater sense of self-confidence. This self-confidence may very well be the element that saves one from harm.

Could you provide an idea of how your day-to-day attitude and approach to living in a modern metropolis changed after you started learning krav maga? *People worldwide look on New York as a tough place to live.*

Born and raised in New York City, I love all it has to offer. The culture, the beauty, and the history draw in thousands of tourists a year who marvel at its magnificence. Like any large city, crime is always a concern. New York is home not only to families, politicians, and stars but also to drug addicts, criminals, and thugs. While caution is my way of life, I often feel vulnerable living in a city that presents so many dangers. Needless to say, today's state of terrorism only exacerbates this concern. My constant vigilance coupled with my knowledge of *krav maga* has made me a stronger woman and, in turn, less of a victim. As I continue to arm myself with the *krav maga's* unparalleled techniques, I am ensuring my own safety in an increasingly dangerous world.

In summary, what would you say are the main benefits that krav maga *training has given you, both physically and mentally?*

Krav maga has helped me reach my best self. Learning how to defend oneself is the most empowering thing one can do. *Krav maga* has given me a stronger body and a sharper mind—not to mention sharper elbows! As a daughter, a sister, and a friend, I feel so fortunate to share my knowledge with my loved ones and others in need of training so that they may feel the security I feel.

Krav maga creator Imi Lichtenfeld has indeed allowed us to, in his own words, "walk in peace." Plus, I believe every girl should know how to throw a good elbow and punch combination!

TRUE KRAVIST

Kim Pimley, a *krav maga* student and mother, responds to a few questions.

What motivated you to take krav maga?

I wanted to learn practical self-defense. *Krav maga* is geared toward surviving an actual confrontation where there are no rules. In addition, as I had hoped, it is excellent fitness training.

How important do you believe it is for women to learn self-defense? Or do you think it is enough to take sensible and safe precautions?

Sensible and safe precautions are a great first step, but they are just plan A. If and when the precautions don't work, you have to be prepared to go to plan B. Years ago, in the seemingly safe confines of a university quadrangle at noon, I was attacked; luckily, I escaped by yelling and running. If the assailant had had a tighter grip or had covered my mouth, I would not have known how to extricate myself. Now I know, and it's very comforting to have increased my chances for survival.

In what way does krav maga *offer a comprehensive approach to the subject of female self-protection?*

Krav maga starts with the assumption that the attacker will be a larger, stronger male. The emphasis is on developing reflexes that both protect your own body as well as attack the vulnerable areas of even the largest and most aggressive assailant. This simultaneous defense and attack allows you to stop the assailant's momentum and create an opportunity to escape.

Continued on next page

Many women don't believe that any self-defense system, including krav maga, *will prevail when faced with a large, physically stronger, and aggressive male. What are your personal feelings and thoughts on this?*

It's simply not true, and worse, it's an abrogation of personal responsibility. Proven techniques exist that give you the means with which to escape and survive an attack by someone twice your size, either unarmed or armed. You owe it to yourself and your family to equip yourself to deal with this threat. Attacks happen everywhere—in suburban malls, office parks, and tree-lined streets, as well as in gritty urban areas. No one is immune.

As a mother, do you feel krav maga *training provides a better sense of family security?*

Our job as parents is to prepare our children spiritually, mentally, and physically to survive and thrive in the world. Whether we like it or not, physical survival isn't just eating well and exercising; it also means self-defense. The don't-talk-to-strangers lecture is only a start; it does not equip children to survive an actual attack. As difficult as it is to imagine your child being attacked, it is irresponsible *not* to imagine it, and to instead leave your child defenseless in the face of danger. *Krav maga* provides tangible escape and defense strategies for the most aggressive attacks, and I'm grateful that my son is learning these important lessons.

Are women more acutely aware of the potential for violence in situations and environments? Can such situational awareness lead to their having the feeling of being a "victim in waiting"? If so, what solutions to this can krav maga *offer?*

I'm a small-framed woman who is often in urban locations around the world, well dressed. If that doesn't say "target", I don't know what does. Admitting this fact is the first step toward effectively managing it, and the next step has been to take sensible precautions. But since precautions don't always work, the final step has been to learn *krav maga*'s defense strategies. Now, because I'm learning to reflexively confront an attack, I no longer have to feel like a "victim in waiting."

> **In summary, what would you say are the main benefits that krav maga *training has given you, both physically and mentally?***
>
> After two years of training, I'm physically much stronger and more focused. While I've always exercised and maintained a healthy weight, lately I hear a lot of "What have you been doing? You are *really* in shape." Awfully nice to hear at forty-six!
>
> More important, I feel mentally prepared. Like any challenges in life—building a business, raising a family, dealing with a setback—it's accomplishable when you have tools and a strategy. I don't have to expend energy worrying and wondering what I would do if I was attacked, because now I know. And that's very empowering.

feel most comfortable with and which give you the greatest confidence. Put just as much emphasis on mental training as you do on the physical. Remember, your mind-set must be to dominate your opponent. Confidence combined with mental and physical ruggedness provide the decided advantage in a violent encounter. Confidence must not, however, lead to overconfidence. *Never underestimate your opponent, and always expect the unexpected.*

In *krav maga*, you will learn a few elementary techniques that you can perform instinctively and adapt to myriad situations. You'll know how to stop and, if necessary, maim an opponent by striking vital points and organs or applying breaking pressure to the attacker's joints.

Range and Distance Reviewed

Range and distance are integral to your self-defense strategy. With *krav maga*, instinctively you will kick an attacker if you feel he is in leg range or elbow him if he is in close proximity. Optimally, you can debilitate your attacker before he can touch you, but such precision and timing are often difficult. If he has already closed the distance and is in physical contact with you, he has entered your medium and close ranges. The following techniques cover your possible ranges from close to medium to long.

Regardless of the type of strike you deliver, remember to shift your body weight forward to deliver your combative strike. That allows you to place all of your body weight behind the combative strike, connecting with greater force. Here are some review pointers for striking effectively:

1. Use your entire body mass by pivoting at the hips and striking through your target.
2. Breathe.
3. Aim for vulnerable targets.

Elbow and Knee Combatives

Your elbows and knees provide some of your most effective and durable personal weapons. The power generated by these short-range combatives, especially in combination, is unparalleled. The key is to turn your hips completely through the strikes and shift your entire body weight through the target. Following are some of the most effective elbow and knee combatives.

Mastering Knees and Elbows

Regardless of your body size or muscular strength, you can deliver powerful strikes with your hands and elbows. The power behind the strike comes from proper execution, not from body size or muscular strength. I often select the largest male in the class to play the part of *uki*—the would-be attacker, more affectionately known as our resident "punching dummy." I then ask Katherina, one of the IKMA's leading female instructors, to convince all who are watching, and especially our *uki*, of *krav maga's* power. Without fail, Kat's powerful kick will send our good-natured target stumbling backward. He also might be taken down with an agonizing wrist lock only to find the heel of Kat's size eight sneaker resting on his throat.

Your strike will generate more force if you accelerate your speed as you extend your limb and put all of your body weight (mass) behind it. This requires proper body positioning and technique. *Krav maga* techniques do not rely on strength. Rather, the system works for anyone, of any shape and size. Elizabeth, who weighs 100 pounds, can easily incapacitate a 250-pound man if she puts all of her 100 pounds behind her strike and aims for a vulnerable target, such as the groin or neck.

Weapons of Opportunity Reviewed

You can use defensive weapons of opportunity and objects of distraction to gain a decisive advantage or level the fighting field. You can distract an opponent simply by spitting into his eyes while simultaneously kicking him in the groin. You can also slip off your high heels and jam a heel into an attacker's eyes. You can throw liquid into his face or an earring to distract him while simultaneously delivering a groin kick or otherwise hobbling him.

Defensive weapons of opportunity can be loosely grouped into six categories:

1. **Blunt objects.** These include sticks, flashlights, stones, chairs, magazines, books, garbage can lids, briefcases, bottles, shoes, and wrenches.
2. **Edged or pointed objects.** These include broken bottles, keys, scissors, pens, forks, and cooking thermometers.
3. **Flexible elongated objects.** These include belts, chains, ropes, jackets, and towels.
4. **Distraction objects and irritant liquids/sprays.** These include keys, coins, watches, loose papers, cellular phones, jewelry, clothing, perfume, spittle, and aerosols. Note that certain liquids or sprays may result in a temporary or even more permanent blinding effect.
5. **Defensive shield-type objects.** These include chairs, briefcases, duffle bags, garbage can lids, and other shieldlike objects.

Elbow Strikes

In this section you'll learn numerous strikes with your elbows. As you deliver an elbow strike, you may keep the hand of the striking arm either open or clenched in a fist. By keeping the hand open, the muscles are less tense before impact, allowing you to tighten them a split second before impact. A clenched fist tightens the forearm and active muscle groups to increase the strength of impact and help prevent injury but may be slightly slower because you expend some energy by tensing your muscles. Use the hand position that is most comfortable for you prior to delivering the elbow strike. You can achieve the best of both worlds by clenching the fist just prior to impact, while the elbow strike is in motion. This accelerates the strike and conserves energy by not tensing your body longer than necessary.

Front and Rear Horizontal Elbow Strikes

This technique uses the extremely hard surface of the elbow to deliver a strong combative. The power and strength behind this strike are unparalleled. The elbow's path follows whatever opening your opponent gives you. Targets usually include the jaw, cheek, throat, and ear.

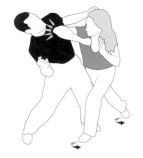

Begin in your left outlet stance with your hands protecting your face. For a front left horizontal elbow, begin to pivot in the direction of the strike on the ball of your left foot, then lower your elbow to begin the combative movement. The hip pivot and transition from arms protecting to your head to the elbow combative are simultaneous. Connect with your target with your front arm parallel to the ground with the hand pressed loosely against your upper chest. Make contact just below the tip of the elbow. As you deliver the front left horizontal elbow, pivot to the right on your front foot in the same direction as the elbow combative so that your front heel nearly faces your target. As you pivot your heel, turn the rest of your body, but keep your eyes on the target. For a rear right elbow strike, pivot to your left on the balls of your feet to deliver the rear strike as illustrated. This rear elbow strike will have more power than your front strike because your hip movement is greater, generating more power. Adjust your rear foot slightly to accommodate your front foot's movement. Keep your rear hand up in a fighting position.

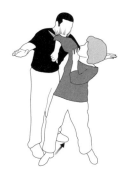

The Rear Horizontal Elbow

Similar to the front horizontal elbow, you'll turn your head to the rear to deliver this strike with your right arm by taking a small step to the rear to open up the hip, allowing you to engage an opponent behind you.

In this strike, your head must lead your body while your hips generate power to deliver this short, compact strike. Bring your wrist into your body with your forearm parallel to the ground. As you turn, use an open-up step with your right leg by stepping to the rear with your rear leg to build momentum and power in the arm delivering the elbow. Begin in your left outlet stance with your hands protecting your face. As you deliver a horizontal elbow with your rear arm, pivot your rear in the same direction as the elbow combative. This will increase the power of the strike. At the same time, move the front foot in the same direction to accommodate the rear foot's movement. Keep your chin tucked.

The Front/Rear Horizontal Elbow Combination

This one-two combination works well together and takes advantage of the momentum of your body movement. This combination is a great tactic to launch into retzev.

Begin in your left outlet stance with your hands protecting your face. Deliver a front horizontal elbow strike. As soon as you reach your maximum left pivot, immediately follow up with a rear horizontal strike. You can also deliver the horizontal elbow strike from a crouch.

The Lateral Elbow

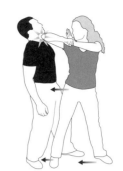

A lateral elbow strike can attack an opponent who is standing to your side. Use this strike to target the face, jaw, and throat. In addition, depending on height and positioning, you can throw a modified horizontal elbow to the opponent's ribs, midsection, kidneys, and other targets of opportunity. This strike is combines well with the horizontal elbow as a follow up combative into retzev.

Practice the technique from either your left outlet stance or a casual stance. Position your striking arm similar to the horizontal elbow starting position. Bring your striking arm parallel to the ground while making a fist and draw your forearm close to your body. As with your other combative strikes, synchronize your lower-and upper-body movements. As you deliver the strike, take a short sidestep forward in the same direction your elbow is traveling. This movement shifts the body weight behind the blow. For a right elbow, step to your right; for a left elbow strike, step to your left. As you step in the direction of your strike, extend the elbow as you make contact using your triceps muscle. With your rear leg, take the same size step as the forward leg, ending in roughly the same equidistant leg position from which you began. Prior to taking the step, bring the hand of your non-striking elbow in front of your face on the same side as the elbowing arm. This covering movement further protects your face and sets you up for your next combative.

The Uppercut Elbow

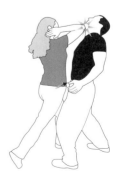

The uppercut elbow can seriously damage your opponent's exposed chin, throat, or groin and works particularly well when the attacker is taller than you.

Stand in the left outlet stance. Bend your knees slightly to generate power from the lower body, allowing your hips to explode through the target. Pivot the front leg inward and straighten your knees as you deliver an upward elbow by bring-ing the striking arm close to your body and thrust your elbow upward close to your front ear for proper follow-through. You may wish to keep your hand open to avoid striking yourself in the ear.

The Perpendicular Rear Elbow

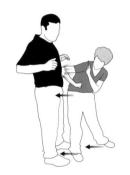

The perpendicular rear elbow delivers a compact strike to an opponent's groin, midsection, face, or other target. In this strike, your hips once again create the power by opening up as you take a short step backward with the leg on the same side. (This strike works well combined with a follow-up groin strike and rear vertical elbow.)

Start in a left or general outlet stance. Keeping your striking arm close to your body, look up and over your shoulder in the di-rection of your strike. Step back slightly with the same-side leg as your striking arm. As you shift your body weight through the strike, make impact with the elbow to the groin. You can keep your hand either open or clenched.

The Rear Vertical Elbow

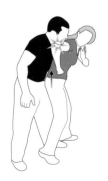

The rear vertical elbow strike is another good follow-on to the short rear elbow targeting the jaw and throat.

Start in the left outlet stance with your legs slightly bent. Make a fist to strengthen your arms and shoulder. Look where you are striking. Then explode upward with your hips, shoulder, and arm, targeting the solar plexus, throat, and face with the top of your elbow.

The Over-the-Top Elbow

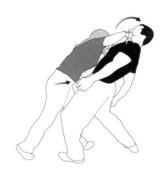

The over-the- top strike is designed to slam down on your opponent. Targets include the brow ridge, nose, ear, and throat. This can be combined strongly with horizontal and uppercut elbows into retzev.

The over-the-top elbow uses a hip pivot movement that's somewhere between those used in the straight punch and roundhouse punch. Beginning from your outlet stance, bring the striking elbow up and over, rotating over the top, from head height to sternum. This strike can be especially effective if you are able to trap one or both of your opponent's arms with your forward arm to negate his defenses. You can also use a weapon to strike over the top; however, your arms should not cross. Instead, they should move in parallel.

The Downward Elbow Strike

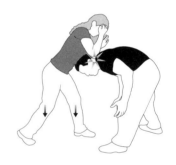

The downward elbow strike is similar to the vertical hammer fist. Targets include the back of the neck, in between the shoulder blades, and the kidneys. If your opponent is on the ground, his face, the back of his neck, and the groin become targets.

From your left outlet stance, execute the same motion as a vertical hammer fist, but this time connect with your elbow. Do not bring your arm higher than you would position it in your general outlet stance.

The Downward Hammer Fist

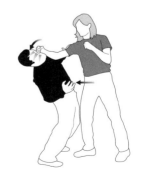

The hammer fist involves using the fleshy part of the closed fist (pinky side) by keeping the knuckles parallel to the ground. The downward hammer fist usually targets the back of the neck but can also be used against the face, groin, kidneys, and in between the shoulder blades, depending on the opponent's position. This also a good strike if you find yourself on the ground.

From your left outlet stance, lower your center of gravity by bending your knees and simultaneously bring your fist down on your target, moving your body in concert. Do not bring your arm higher than you would position it in your regular outlet stance. A weapon can be brought down on a target in the same way.

PERFECTING YOUR ELBOW TECHNIQUES

Shadow elbowing can enhance your striking skills and fluidity. Practice without any contact. Methods include the following:

1. Use a mirror to practice elbow combinations from both left and right outlet stances.
2. Move in and out with elbow, using proper footwork.
3. Close your eyes to perform combinations as you envision elbow combinations and movements.

Attacking Sensitive Areas

In addition to punching and elbowing your opponent, you can also use your fingers, thumbs, and many other parts of your upper body to inflict a great amount of damage, especially if you target vulnerable areas such as the eyes, groin, and fingers. Although simple to learn and execute, the techniques in this section will become a valuable part of your *krav maga* arsenal.

Groin Strike with the Hand

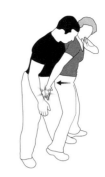

A highly effective follow-up strike to the perpendicular rear elbow or an independent strike in its own right. Use this strike to target one of the body's most sensitive targets. A vertical rear elbow is a good follow-up to launch into retzev.

To strike the groin with your hand, cup your hand. You may strike forward, to the side, or the rear by keeping the fingertips down toward the ground. By whipping your hand into the groin, you create a potent debilitating blow. You can also use a hammer fist, by clenching the fingers into a fist, for more power. You can also attack an opponent's groin in the same way by cupping your hand and striking with the palm out.

Palm Heel Strike

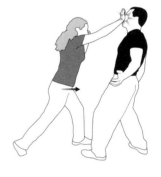

When using this direct and fast strike, aim for the nose or jaw. Similar to straight punches in footwork, weight redistribution, and chin positioning, the palm heel strike is an effective intermediate-range strike, particularly for those who are not confident in the strength of their wrists and fists to execute regular punches. Elbows and knees are good follow-ups to launch into retzev.

Starting from your regular outlet stance, make a palm heel by tightly curling your fingers and pressing your thumb close to your hand. Bend your fingers toward your shoulder, exposing your palm. Your knuckles should be facing upward. Pivot your right leg slightly onto the ball of the foot as you drive your hips, rear shoulder, and arm forward toward your target. Tuck your chin into your right shoulder to protect it from an incoming strike. You can combine this technique with the next technique to rake the eyes.

Eye Gouges

Finger strikes to the eyes can disable an opponent quickly and effectively. The eyeball can be collapsed with minimum pressure. Blinding or partially blinding an attacker sets up retzev *follow-up strikes to end a confrontation quickly.*

For a multiple-finger strike, fold your fingers slightly inward toward your palm and spread them just enough so they do not touch. This will reduce the possibility of injuring them on impact. If the impact is hard, flexing the fingers inward will collapse them into their natural articulation. Note that the fingers are fragile and can easily be fractured even when taking precautions. Execute the strike with a body movement similar to your straight punches, with the fingers making contact with the eyes.

You can also strike the eyes with your thumbs, penetrating the eye socket. Use your opponent's cheekbone as a guide. A rule of thumb (pardon the pun): if you can find the cheekbone, you can find the eye. This is particularly important if you are not in a position to see your attacker, such as a ground-fighting situation or if it is dark. You can insert one or both of your thumbs into your opponent's eye sockets.

Stomp

If you knock the attacker to the ground while you are still standing, the stomp is a simple and highly effective combative targeting the top of the attacker's foot or other exposed areas such as the groin, throat, ribs, or hands. You can also strike his Achilles tendon if he is kneeling; this will likely hobble him.

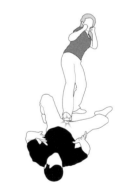

You must make contact to the targeted area with your heel by lifting your foot upward.

Front Straight Offensive Kick

Kicking with your rear leg will connect with enormous power to your opponent's knee, groin, abdomen, and midsection. Higher targets include the neck and the head. Elbows and hammer fists are strong follow-up combatives into retzev.

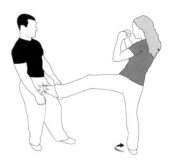

From your left outlet stance, take the longest possible step forward with your right leg to practice the movement. As you step, turn out your left foot approximately 90 degrees. Notice how your body elongates and your non-kicking left base leg naturally pivots out, with your toes pointed to your left. (Although the optimal turn is 90 degrees, some people experience knee discomfort when they turn the knee this far.) Turning out your front leg will thrust the hips of your base (rear) leg forward, giving you maximum extension and power using *glicha*, sliding step, to carry your body weight through the kick. This enables you to throw your body mass behind the kick.

Launch the kick from low to high, to make it harder for your opponent to pick it up visually. Connect with the ball of your foot against your target. Do not raise the knee up and then push out to kick. Rather, snap or thrust the kick toward the target. After impact, land with your kicking leg forward. Keep your hands up the entire time. Many people unconsciously drop their hands to improve their balance.

Note: You can practice keeping your hands up by grabbing your shirt collar as you kick.

The Rear Straight Offensive Kick

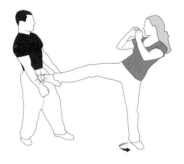

You'll use similar kicking and base leg movements for the rear kick as you did for the front kick to maximize your reach and kicking power. Elbows and hammer fists are strong follow-up combatives into retzev.

From your left outlet stance, take the largest step you can with your left leg and remain in that position. You will notice how your body elongates again and your non-kicking base leg pivots in approximately a 90-degree angle with your toes pointed to your right. Whip your front leg out as though your are thrusting the ball of your foot through a target, again from low to high. As you kick, keep your hands up to protect your head. To enhance your footwork and balance, learn to deliver the kick and then retreat back into an opposite fighting stance. As your kicking leg touches the ground, use the retreating footwork you learned with your straight punches to move your body backward.

LOWER BODY DRILLS

To familiarize yourself with lower-body techniques, practice the following drill. Substitute any lower-body technique you wish to learn for the straight kick.

1. From the left outlet stance: 20 kicks with the forward (left) leg and 20 kicks with the rear (right) leg, pivoting correctly on the base leg while simultaneously placing the hands in the correct fighting position.
2. From the right outlet stance: 20 kicks with the forward (right) leg and 20 kicks with the rear (left) leg, pivoting correctly on the base leg while simultaneously placing the hands in the correct fighting position.
3. From the left outlet stance: 20 right/left switching kick combinations, pivoting correctly on the respective base legs while simultaneously placing the hands in the correct fighting position.
4. From the right outlet stance: 20 left/right switching kick combinations, pivoting correctly on the respective base legs while simultaneously placing the hands in the correct fighting position.

Straight Kick When on the Ground

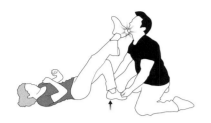

Even when you're on the ground, you can successfully launch a front straight kick against an opponent who is standing.

As you fall to the ground, protect your head, using similar arm positioning to your outlet stance to form your defensive posture. Although you may periodically drop your arms to the ground to move your body away from your opponent or rotate your body to meet a threat from a different angle, keep your arms in a protective position for your head as often as you can. As you kick, keep your base leg against the ground for leverage. Thrust out the kick with your other leg. Use your upper back and shoulders as a launching platform, allowing your torso to lift off the ground, putting its weight behind the kick. Make contact with either the heel or ball of your foot and recoil quickly to avoid having your leg caught by your opponent. Launching this kick from the ground becomes an offensive movement, due to your angle of attack against a standing opponent.

Straight Knees

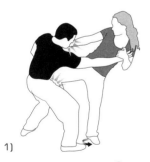

1)

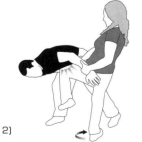

2)

Once you know how to straight-kick, you know how to straight-knee. Knee attacks provide some of the most punishing strikes and are a strong finish to any technique. Elbows and hammerfists are strong follow-up combatives into retzev.

Knee your opponent with the same technique you use to kick. Rather than make contact with your foot, however, you'll thrust your kneecap into your target. By returning to your left outlet stance, you will rechamber your knee which provides additional powerful and debilitating strikes.

SIDE KICK AND SIDE KICK
WHILE ON THE GROUND

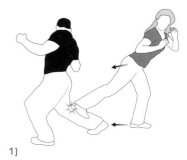

1)

The side kick enables you to kick a threat to your side or rear and is one of your most formidable striking weapons against the attacker's forward knee, thighs, or midsection. The sidekick also works well if you find yourself on the ground with your attacker standing over you. The attacker's knees, thighs, and groin usually present the best targets when in this position. If opportune, you can also increase the effectiveness of this combative by hooking the attacker's heel with your lower leg to immobilize the knee just prior to impact, thereby increasing the trauma to the knee.

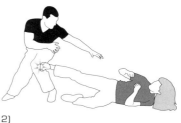

2)

By varying your outlet stance or "cheating"—positioning your feet almost perpendicular to your opponent—the side kick can target an opponent in front of you. Execute the side kick with your front leg, which is closer to your target. Once again, pivoting and aligning the base leg in the appropriate direction is essential to maximize reach and power. To execute the standing kick, raise your front kicking leg until your leg is bent 90 degrees and your thigh is parallel to the ground. Deliver the kick by thrusting your raised leg out, pointing the heel toward the target and curling the toes toward your body. Keep your foot parallel with the ground as you make contact. As with every other kick, your body weight must shift forward into your target.

To execute the kick while on the ground, keep both hands raised in a defensive posture and one leg on the ground. Kick sideways in an upward motion, curling your toes toward you and connecting with your heel. You may wish to place one forearm on the ground to establish a strong kicking base with good balance. Keep your non-kicking leg flush against the ground prior to the kick. As you kick, this base leg may rise slightly off the ground to give you leverage.

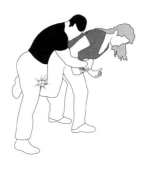

Mule Kick

Another highly effective kick, the mule kick, uses an upward kicking motion with your heel to connect with your opponent's groin when he is standing behind you in close proximity. Vertical and horizontal elbows are good retzev *transitions that allow you to turn and face your opponent.*

From your regular left outlet stance, shift your body weight over one leg and kick up with the leg that is between your attacker's legs, as if you were going to kick yourself in the buttock. Deliver the strike with an upward arcing motion and hit the most opportune target, including the shin, groin, and abdomen.

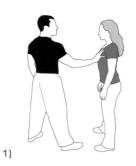
1)

Chest Grab Defenses

These defenses build on previous defenses attacking your assailant's vulnerable areas, including the eyes, throat, groin, midsection, and knees.

Chest Grab from the Front

You have the option of pinning your attacker's hand(s) to your body with one of your arms while attacking his eyes, throat, and groin, followed by secondary strikes into full-blown *retzev*.

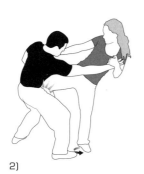
2)

Chest Grab with Assailant's Arm Draped over the Shoulder

If the assailant drapes his arm around your shoulder while standing next to you, you may use a variation of the headlock from the side as a defense. The headlock defense reaches around the attacker's torso with your left hand to gouge his eye and slap his groin with your right hand. Alternatively, you can pluck the hand away with your same-side hand and slap him in the groin with your other hand. Continue to attack, using knuckle-edge strikes to the throat, knees, and other *retzev* combatives.

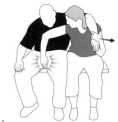

1)

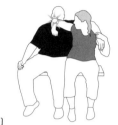

2)

Note: Variations of these defenses can be used when seated. In addition to strikes, another seated defense is available if an assailant places his hand on one of your legs. Clamp down your left hand on his hand and attack his elbow with an armbar or break by thrusting the blade of your left forearm against above his elbow. You will drive him forward out of his seat and can continue your retzev *counterattack.*

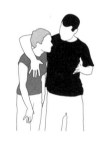

1)

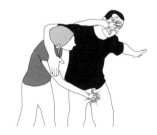

2)

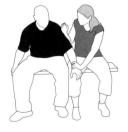

1)

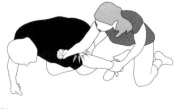

2)

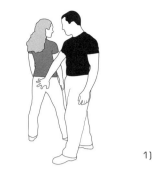

1)

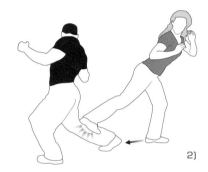

2)

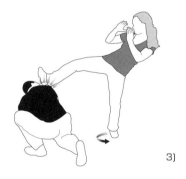

3)

Buttocks Grab Defense

This powerful defense involves a rear kick to the assailant's knee.

If an assailant is walking past you or is behind you and makes hand contact with your buttocks, you can deliver a powerful rear kick to his knee using your heel. If he is passing you, you will likely have to use *glicha* (a sliding step backward on the ball of your left foot, as shown in the illustration) to collapse his knee. Once your assailant is down, you have additional options to begin your *retzev* counterattack, such as stomping on his exposed Achilles tendon, additional kicks to the kidneys and head, punches to the neck, elbows, and other options. If he comes from directly behind you and is facing your back, the same rear kick may be employed, or you can execute rear elbows followed by *retzev*. Note that a kick to the bend of the knee will most likely collapse it with minimal damage, while a kick to the side or front of the knee can cause extensive damage.

Your knees and the balls of your feet (especially when clad in shoes) serve as hard and durable striking surfaces and are the most powerful fighting weapons that you can use at maximum fighting range. When you kick or knee your opponent, you engage your body's largest muscle groups, including the gluteus, quadriceps, and hamstrings. As with punching, if you put your entire body mass and strength behind your kick or knee, you can deliver a devastating blow, no matter your size or weight.

You can perform *krav maga* kicks at low, medium, and head-level heights. To execute high kicks, you'll need a high degree of flexibility, as well as enough strength in your outer thighs to lift your leg. For most kicks, you'll make contact with the ball of your foot. To accustom your feet to striking, curl your toes up toward you and repeatedly tap the ground with the ball of your foot. Increase the force of your taps as you become more comfortable with this foot positioning. To strike with your heel for a stomp, arc your toes toward your knee to expose the heel. Perform the same tapping exercise to accustom your heel to striking.

Note that this heel exercise is a combative kick in itself, known as the stomp, which is useful when an opponent is on the ground and you are standing.

The sidekick and rear defensive kick build your arsenal of combatives, enabling you to kick a threat to your side or rear. The side kick and rear defensive kicks will become some of your most formidable striking weapons. The side kick is highly effective against lateral attacks against you, such as straight punches, as you can use the kick's superior reach and power against the attacker's forward knee, thighs, or midsection.

For all straight kicks and knees, think of your kneecap as a directional finder or pointer. Wherever the knee is pointed, the kick or knee will follow. Hip alignment is paramount to keeping your leg on target.

Note: Do not fully extend the kicking leg unless you are impacting a target. Rather, only extend about 90 percent. As with punches, you can hyperextend your knee by locking the joint.

Release from a Pull from Behind Covering the Mouth

An assailant can attack from behind by covering your mouth with one hand and strong-arming you with his other hand. This type of attack often involves pulling you backward. Your defense is straightforward: plucking the attacker's hand covering your mouth and performing a wrist release to disengage your other arm.

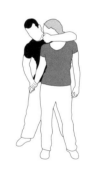

1)

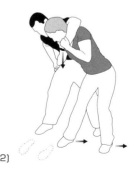

2)

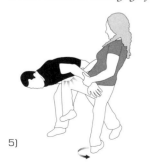

5)

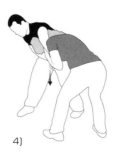

4)

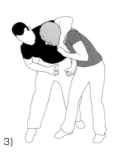

3)

You must move with the attacker's pull. Pluck his hand from your mouth while turning your right shoulder into him by stepping back with the right leg. Simultaneously release your left hand from his grip by sliding it across his body, creating an opening where his pointer and thumb meet. As you clear his body, follow with knee strikes and other *retzev* counterattacks.

Basic Ground Defenses for Women Against Assault

Using the Brakes to Disengage from an Attacker

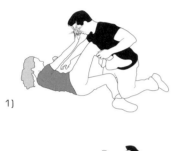

1)

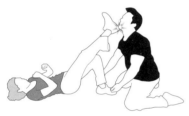

2)

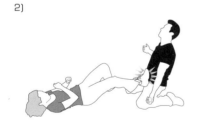

3)

The "brakes" technique disengages you from an attacker who is trying to spread your legs or mount you. Eye gouges, throat strikes, palm heels, and additional kicks are strong follow-up combatives.

By turning on your side, you can use your top shin and knee to keep an attacker at bay as you deliver combatives such as eye gouges and throat strikes. Remember, your hips and legs are your most powerful muscles. As you separate yourself from your attacker you will likely gain the opportunity to kick him with both legs in the groin or head using a straight or side kick, in either case striking with the heel. Get up as quickly as you can by sliding your left leg back and onto the ball of your foot while posting one hand on the ground, to deliver more combatives and make your escape. While engaged in the brace, you may also use your left leg to kick his groin with your heel or kick his thigh to knock him to the ground, allowing you to get in additional combative kicks in order to make an escape.

Side Shimmy to Disengage from an Attacker

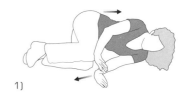

1)

Similar to the brakes, the side shimmy is another technique that disengages you from an attacker who is trying to spread your legs or mount you. Eye gouges and throat strikes are good combatives to create separation from your attacker.

Once again, by turning on your side, you can use your most powerful lower-body muscle groups to keep an attacker at bay as you deliver combative kicks. Once you separate yourself from your attacker, you will likely gain the opportunity to kick him in the groin or head using a straight kick or side kick on the ground. Make contact with your heel. Get up by sliding your left leg back and onto the ball of your foot while posting one hand on the ground, to deliver more combatives and make your escape.

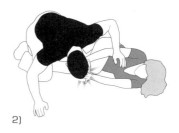

2)

Counterattacks When the Attacker Is Between Your Legs (the Guard)

These powerful counterattack options are designed to hurt your attacker. A woman's more flexible hip structure makes these techniques particularly effective. Eye gouges and throat strikes are good initiators to disable your opponent.

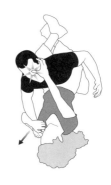

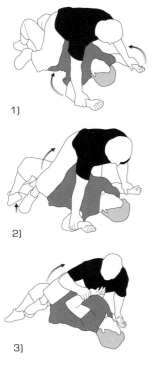

1)

2)

3)

4)

Release when Attacker Has Pinned Your Hands to the Ground While Straddling You

This release allows you to escape an attacker's attempt to pin your arms to the ground with his full body weight holding you down.

This technique can be executed while an attacker is mounted on top of you or between your legs and pinning your arms. If the attacker is mounted, bring your elbows sharply and directly to your side while turning to your right side by bridging on your right shoulder and balls of the feet to hip-buck or launch the attacker to your left. It is very important that you slide your elbows to your side and bridge your hips at the same time. Your attacker is likely to have all of his weight on your hands and fall forward as you throw him off balance. There is the danger of his delivering an inadvertent head butt to you, so you should protect your face by turning it to the side you are bridging your opponent. Immediately attack the groin and other vulnerable areas.

Choke Release from the Ground with the Attacker Straddling You

If an attacker chokes you from a straddling position (also known as the mounted position), he'll be able to push his upper body down on your throat, creating greater pressure. You can still, however, extricate yourself from this seemingly grim situation.

Tuck your chin, yank down on the attacker's right hand just below the thumb joint, and attack his left eye with a thumb gouge to the inside of his choking arms while turning to your left side to buck him from you by turning on your left shoulder and

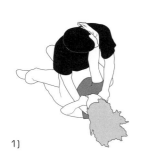

1)

balls of the feet to launch the attacker. To buck your hips, you must raise them up and to one side to throw the attacker. Practice this buck by lying flat on the ground with your legs bent and feet on the ground. Rotate your body to one side by raising one shoulder off the ground, transferring your weight to your other shoulder. Your feet will move to accommodate your turning movement. You should be able to launch the attacker provided he has not hooked his heels into your sides. Once you have thrown him, you are in a strong position to hit your opponent repeatedly in the groin. If you cannot launch him, attack with strikes to the groin, midsection, neck, and face along with elbows to his thighs, launching him whenever and however you can.

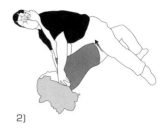

2)

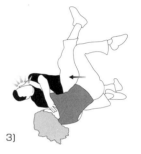

3)

Choke Release from the Ground with the Attacker Between Your Legs in the Guard

Use this defense if an attacker tries to choke you when positioned between your legs while on his knees (or if he is attempting to position himself there). You can employ this technique before the attacker attempts to grab your neck. You can also use it to defend against a sexual assault.

Tuck your chin. Pluck the attacker's hand just below the thumb to remove it from your throat while bridging on your shoulder to deliver an eye gouge or throat strike in between his arms. Do not counterattack to the outside because he can block this move by moving his arm out to defend. Once you have released, slide to the brakes position by pressing one knee into his torso. Disengage and kick the assailant with a side kick or heel kick to the head. Continue with various strikes as openings present themselves. Escape as soon as possible.

An upright arm bar variation against the attacker's right arm (or left arm) may be executed by swinging over your left leg (right leg for the left arm bar) and isolating the attacker's arm by wrapping your leg around his right shoulder (left shoulder for the left arm bar). Your other leg will be under the armpit of his free arm. Once the arm is secured, extend your hips to apply breaking pressure to the arm.

Release from an Attacker Smothering You with a Pillow

If an attacker attempts to suffocate you with a pillow from a straddling position or mounted position or from a side position, he'll be able to push his upper body down on your nose and mouth, preventing you from breathing. You can still, however, extricate yourself from this seemingly grim situation.

This is a bad situation, but you must not panic. If you are lying on your back, you must immediately turn your head to the side to create an air pocket while dislodging the attacker's hands. Your correct instinct will be to turn on your side to escape. You must either pluck his hands by yanking down where his wrist meets his hand or remove his hands from your face by forcefully "swimming" over the top with your free arm as you turn on your side. The goal is to dislodge both of the attacker's arms or catch both of them under your armpit and keep moving to thwart the suffocation attempt. Clear the pillow from your face to draw breath and keep fighting. Do not turn facedown under any circumstances because of the extreme difficulty in defending against this dire situation. If an attacker came from the side of the bed and attempted the smother, the technique is similar except the attacker does not have a mount on you. If you are lying on your stomach, you must not allow the attacker to force your head into the mattress to suffocate you. In that case, keep your head turned to the side to draw breath. Similar to the drowning defense, pluck his hands or clear his hands by bringing your bicep to your ear and forearm to the top of your head while turning in the direction of your other shoulder with all your might. Covers and sheets are likely to hinder your lower-body counterattacks. You must create space from the attacker and free your lower body for kicks and knees. Of course, you should use any weapons of opportunity.

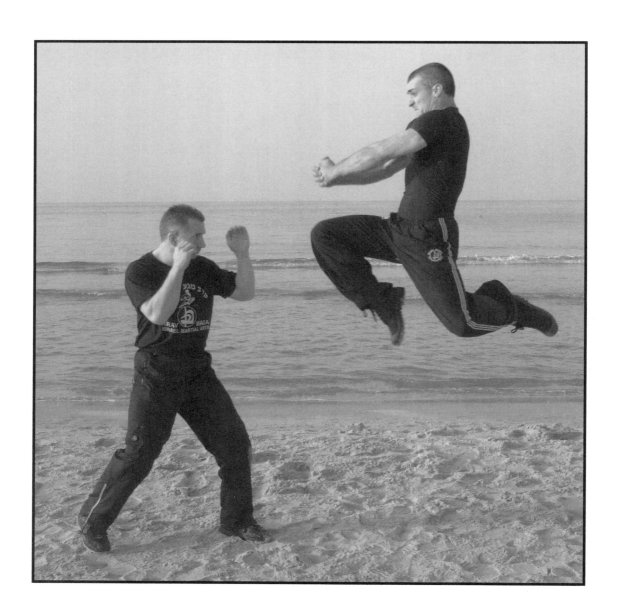

CHAPTER 9

The Kravist Training Plan

Welcome to the advanced *kravist* training plan, a twelve-week program designed to take your fighting ability and fitness to the next level. For this program you will continue to practice the *krav maga* techniques for a recommended four to five hours a week, spread over three or four days. Some of your practice sessions will include a partner, while others you can complete alone. For most individual practice and conditioning sessions, I recommend you complete your drills in front of a mirror. With dedication and practice, you will advance quickly. While it requires many years of study to become an expert under the Israeli curriculum, you can achieve street skill effectiveness against unarmed confrontations with shocking and gratifying speed.

TRUE KRAVIST

I asked my friend and *krav maga* enthusiast Doug Bercume, a professional strength and conditioning coach and professor at Oakland University, to add his insights into *krav maga* conditioning:

"*Krav maga* is the ultimate combined dynamic application of functional power, strength, speed and agility. *Krav maga* is based on natural (proper) joint mechanics to harness all of an individual's musculature and weight into each combative. Proper strength and conditioning are essential to enhancing one's ability to train for ballistic combat.

"Most important, *krav maga* emphasizes realistic training. Specific strength and conditioning for *krav maga* are no different than in any other athletic pursuit. *Krav maga* requires power (speed times strength), agility, dynamic flexibility, and aerobic and all-important anaerobic conditioning. To be effective, the training must be multiplanar and multidirectional, and occur at velocities similar to combat scenarios. Therefore, dynamic movement patterns are preferred over traditional, single-muscle-group methods.

"All good strength and conditioning programs emphasize injury prevention while developing the desired strength and agility response. Stability, flexibility, and muscle balance are vital to preventing injuries. The central nervous system will not allow your muscles to produce muscular force beyond the stability of your joints. Poor stability results in a lack of power. A lack of flexibility can prevent the proper execution and application of various combative techniques. Both deficiencies may result in a loss of power or injury. Developing and maintaining proper core strength, stability, and flexibility is the nexus of our *kravist* conditioning program.

"Once there is a sound level of core strength, stability, and flexibility, strength and power can then be effectively trained. Traditional strength training focuses primarily on absolute strength (how much you can bench-press). Absolute strength, however, is not the key to most sports-specific training effectiveness. Functional strength is defined as the degree of strength you can apply during a real movement at high velocity. As such, functional strength is the most important type of strength needed for ballistic combatives. *Krav maga*'s techniques are equally effective for men and women because they utilize biomechanically advantageous movements and emphasize the functional application of strength, not strength alone.

"We focus on two types of power: speed-strength and strength-speed. Speed-strength is the ability to move a light object quickly (e.g. hands, feet, elbows, knees), such as when practicing upper- and lower-body combatives. Strength-speed is the ability to move a heavy object quickly (e.g., another person), such as when practicing clinches, throws, and takedowns. Both types of power are important and require different types of training.

"While *krav maga* is designed to take an opponent down quickly and is not designed for fighting rounds in the ring, depending on the fight situation you may require a high level of anaerobic endurance to fight at high intensities for long periods of time. The ability to explosively and continuously counterattack requires specific conditioning, much of which can be gained through *krav maga* training itself. *Retzev* training is the prime example of this. Continuous, powerful, unscripted counterattacks to overwhelm your opponent, when done regularly, will enhance one's anaerobic capacity. Other methods of interval-type training can be used to train the physiological systems responsible for anaerobic endurance."

Your Warm-up and Cool-down

Warm up before every practice session. Preparing the muscles, joints, and respiratory and circulatory systems for any vigorous activity is essential. First, you should increase your blood flow and heart rate with modest cardiovascular activity such as a light run, riding an exercise bike, jumping jacks, or the like for a minimum of ten minutes. After you warm up, stretch gently to prepare your muscles, ligaments, and tendons for quick explosive movements and maximum extension.

Allow your body to gradually adjust to exertion and strain. Begin with stretching your neck and work your way down the body to your ankles and toes. Make sure to stretch each muscle group. Hold each stretch for a count of ten, using "one one-thousand, two one thousand . . . ten one thousand." Repeat each stretch on the left and right sides of your body.

Training Solo

Practicing techniques without making contact with a pad or person develops muscle memory and conditioning through repetitive movement. But you must also practice the techniques with pad work and partners. Developing and practicing your movements in front of a mirror is one of the best methods to acquire correct form and fluidity. Observing yourself in a mirror will improve your movements and keep your head sighted toward your opponent.

Advanced Balance Exercises

Practicing balance exercises with your eyes open and closed before your *krav maga* training session will improve your coordination and body control. At first keep your hands extended out to your sides for maximum balance. As your balance improves, position your hands in your outlet stance. Extending your arms when kicking is a common mistake that telegraphs your movements to your opponent (always keep your arms up in your outlet stance) and leaves you vulnerable to counterattack. Your center of gravity is just below your navel, so if you begin to lose your balance, drop your hips to lower your center of gravity.

Here are a few exercises to practice:

1. Perform calf raises standing on the balls of your feet, first with your eyes open and then with them closed.
2. Raise one leg, extend it forward, and grab it with the same-side hand, first with your eyes open and then with them closed.
3. Balance from your extended straight knee position and

then your roundhouse knee position with one leg in the air, first keeping your eyes open and then with them closed.

4. Come into an airplane position with one leg extended, one leg raised behind, and your arms spread out to the side, keeping your eyes closed.

5. Complete *retzev* movements for several minutes with your eyes closed to practice your balance, combatives form, fluidity, and stamina. This develops your awareness in addition to your balance.

Coordination Drills

A number of coordination drills will further enhance and develop your fighting capabilities. Your brain is being trained to extend commands to your body to hone both gross and fine motor skills. Here are a few exercises to practice:

1. Perform twenty-five jumping jacks in a normal fashion, but then modify them by:
   a. Your left arm moving rising up and down pointing forward, with your right arm rising up and down and pointing out to the side.
   b. Your right arm moving rising up and down pointing forward, with your left arm rising up and down pointing out to the side.
   c. Your left arm moving in a forward circle and your right arm moving in a reverse circle.
   d. Your right arm moving in a forward circle and your left arm moving in a reverse circle.

2. Shuffle steps forward with arms moving forward. Try to coordinate the left arm moving forward with the left leg and vice versa for the right. Then modify this movement to include:

a. Your left arm moving rising up and down pointing forward, with your right arm rising up and down pointing out to the side.

b. Your right arm moving rising up and down pointing forward, with your left arm rising up and down pointing out to the side.

c. Your left arm moving in a forward circle with your right arm moving in a reverse circle.

d. Your right arm moving in a forward circle with your left arm moving in a reverse circle.

3. Perform a finger coordination drill using your left hand, then your right hand, and then both hands simultaneously. With your left hand, touch your thumb to your pinky and then touch each subsequent finger, moving up the hand from pinky to pointer. With your right hand, touch your thumb to your pointer and then touch each subsequent finger moving "down" hand. When the two hands perform together, your left hand should begin with thumb to pinky while your right hand begins thumb to pointer. The idea is to move the fingers in opposite directions with both hands at the same time to develop coordination.

Advancing Along the Punch Line

This drill is designed to perfect your linear footwork as you move in and out to counterattack. Choose a line on the floor. It can be a floorboard line, a carpet seam, a string you lay down, or whatever else will serve the purpose. Position your fighting stance so that the line bisects your body. Execute left/right and right/left straight punch combinations, advancing and retreating, while maintaining the line in the center of your body. Make sure that your feet move together, covering the same distance in addition to advancing along the punch line.

Shadow Boxing in Front of a Mirror

Practice your striking combinations from chapter 3—from both the left and right outlet stance, using all manners and combinations of punches and elbows—in front of a mirror. In essence, you are your opponent in the mirror. Watch for good form and repeat a movement if you observe yourself incorrectly performing a technique. Be careful not to hyperextend your elbows.

Retzev Exercise Bar Striking Drills

This drill makes use of a weighted bar, commonly found in a gym, or any other type of elongated object that you can wield effectively for a highly effective improvised weapon. I suggest using the lightest-weight bar you can find at first and then progressing gradually to higher weights. You will perform real combat motions with the bar, simulating your upper-body combatives, particularly elbow combatives. You must have adequate space to practice and to avoid injuring anyone else. Proper hip pivoting is essential. This is a superb drill to test if you are following through with your hips when performing combatives by executing them on the balls of your feet. The weight of the bar will also give you a total body workout bonus, both aerobic and anaerobic.

Here is a sample list of bar combatives to practice from your left outlet stance, holding the bar with the forward hand thumb away and rear hand thumb toward your torso. Grip the bar a little wider than shoulder width, leaving substantial room on both ends of the bar to strike an imaginary or heavy bag target. Note that the bar can tear a heavy bag open. Should you decide to beat up a tree, be careful because of reverberations through your practice tool. A word to the wise: the bag and tree usually win. Make sure to turn your hips through each strike while maintaining a firm grip on the bar.

1. **Left horizontal strike** targeting the opponent's head and neck. Pivot on the ball of your left (forward) foot

and on your right (rear) foot to accommodate the left pivot while keeping your head on a swivel to face your target.

2. **Right horizontal strike** targeting the opponent's head and neck. Pivot on the ball of your right (rear) foot and slightly on the ball of your left (front) foot to accommodate the right pivot while keeping your head on a swivel to face your target.

3. **Left uppercut strike** targeting the opponent's groin, midsection, or neck and head (depending on the height of impact you choose). Pivot on the ball of your left (forward) foot and slightly on your right (rear) foot to accommodate the left pivot. Your left hip should turn into your target.

4. **Right uppercut strike** targeting the opponent's groin, midsection, or neck and head (depending on the height of impact you choose.) Pivot on the ball of your right (rear) foot.

5. **Left over-the-top strike** targeting the opponent's head and neck. Pivot on the ball of your left (forward) foot and slightly on your right (rear) foot to accommodate the left pivot while keeping your head on a swivel to face your target. Essentially, you are slashing down on your target. Your right foot will draw back, pulling your hips with it, to allow the bar to come through. Be careful not to smash yourself in the knee.

6. **Right over-the-top strike** targeting the opponent's head and neck. Pivot on the ball of your right (rear) foot, rotating the bar over the top. Do not cross your hands. Keep them firmly grasping the bar. Essentially, you are slashing down on your target using the butt end of the stick. (Note: You can step forward with your right foot after delivering the blow to deliver a thrust at the attacker's head with the same end of the bar.)

7. **Left forward thrust** targeting the opponent's groin, midsection, or neck and head, depending on the height of impact you choose. This movement is similar to your advancing left punch. Move your feet together covering the same distance and thrust forward toward your target. This is a great opening move for your *retzev* bar salvo.

8. **Two-handed blunt thrust** targeting the opponent's head and neck. This movement is similar to an advancing rear straight punch. You will make impact with the section of the bar between your two hands. Move your feet together and shift your entire body weight through the strike.

9. **Lateral left and right thrusts** targeting the opponent's groin, midsection, or neck and head, depending on the height of impact you choose. This movement is similar to your lateral elbows. Strike with the bar as you shift your weight by moving your feet together covering the same distance.

10. **Rear horizontal strikes** targeting the opponent's head and neck. This movement is similar to your rear horizontal elbows. Remember that the head must lead the body; you must turn to see your target before striking. Open up the same-side hip to allow the bar to move through the strike while also generating power.

11. **Rear straight thrusts** targeting the opponent's groin or midsection. This movement is similar to your perpendicular rear elbows. Step back slightly with the same-side leg as the strike. Shift your weight through the strike.

12. As with upper-body combatives, **combine each of these in a logical *retzev* attack**. One example: left horizontal strike, right horizontal strike, left over-the-top strike, left forward thrust, right rear uppercut, finishing with a two-handed blunt thrust.

Training Drills with a Partner

You'll need a training partner to put the techniques into realistic action. Training with multiple partners is beneficial because no two people move exactly alike or have the same capabilities. A partner with longer limbs will attack and defend differently than someone with shorter limbs. Working with different attackers will improve your reactions. Men and women should train with each other interchangeably. Build a mutual working relationship with a number of partners.

You should coordinate training with your partner to ensure maximum training benefit. Designate who will perform the specific technique against the corresponding mock attack. After concrete practice and familiarity with a given technique, series of techniques, and overall training concept, introduce variations.

Effective pad work requires you to work in coordination with your partner. (A heavy bag can be stabilized by your partner but also serves as a good solo training tool.) With pad work, your partner determines your strike combinations by holding the kicking pad or hand pads in a certain manner. For example, if your partner holds his arms straight out with the front of the pads facing you, he is signaling for half-roundhouse punches and forearm strikes. If your partner turns the pads inward so that his palms face each other, he is signaling for chops. If the pads are held with the narrower sides facing you, they are positioned for web strikes. With practice, your partner will meet your strikes mid-motion with the pad.

As you strike through the pad using all of your body mass, emphasize strong hip and shoulder movements. Drive your attacks directly through the target. Use proper footwork to move in and out, especially when leading your forward arm with straight punches. Partners using all-strike padwork should work in concert; the pad holder may begin to move the hand pads and deliver counterattacks when the other partner leaves himself unprotected.

Punching Drills

In and Out Drill

With a partner, you will use timing to exchange punches without making contact. Footwork is essential to move in and out properly and keep the correct distance to avoid any contact with your partner. Remember to keep your feet moving together and covering the same distance as you move in and out. Be sure to use proper hip pivots. Use the following combinations from the left outlet stance (left foot forward):

1. Front/rear straight punches with proper advance and retreat
2. Rear/front straight punches with proper advance and retreat
3. Front/rear straight punches and left/right half-roundhouse punches with proper advance and retreat
4. Combinations of the above such as:
   a. Front straight punch and rear half-roundhouse with proper advance and retreat
   b. Front half-roundhouse and straight rear punch with proper advance and retreat

Line Retzev

Line *retzev* using hands and feet together (Hebrew: *yadim ve reglaim*) is a drill that allows both partners to work freely with each another, practicing their own *krav maga* preferences with open training modalities. *Retzev* is your continuous flow of *krav maga* techniques that allow you to finish the fight. Your opponent has little room for defensive action or counterattack. Upper-body and lower-body combatives become seamless and automatic, pistonlike. For example, as you deliver a straight left half-roundhouse kick, before your foot touches the ground you are already moving into a straight left punch. As soon as you begin to retract your left arm, you deliver a right punch. As your right fist makes impact you are already setting your body in motion for a right half-roundhouse knee.

The drill positions two partners facing one another with an invisible line separating them that they will not cross. Both partners will launch into their individual *retzev* while watching the other. Subconsciously, each partner will perform his individualized continuous combat motion while visualizing the defenses he would perform against his partner's mock attacks. This is a more advanced version of the *retzev* watching drill where one partner remains placid as the other partner performs *retzev* again without making any contact. A more advanced version of the drill is to mirror or duplicate the attacks of your partner, building observation skills and coordination.

Upper-body Combatives

These drills focus on specific punch defenses from chapter 3. Your partner will hold the pad at the correct angle. Be careful to use correct form, paying particular attention not to hyperextend your elbows or misalign your wrists. You will find these drills repeated in different formats in the twelve-week *kravist* training plan that follows. Practice the following combatives from both the left and right outlet stances.

1. Holding the pad straight for a direct attack, 15 repetitions of:
   a. Front half-roundhouse punch
   b. Rear half-roundhouse punch
   c. Straight front forearm strike
   d. Straight rear forearm strike
   e. High forearm strike to the throat
   f. Whipping blows
   g. Combinations using these strikes

2. Holding the pad sideways to allow the edge to be used to simulate the throat, 15 repetitions of:

a. Front straight web strike to the throat

b. Rear straight web strike to the throat

c. Combinations using web strikes to the throat

3. Holding the pad sideways for the proper angle of attack, 15 repetitions of:

a. Inward chop

b. Outward chop

c. Inward and outward chop combinations

Punch Defense Drills

These drills focus on specific punch defenses from chapter 3. For these movements, make sure you and your partner properly execute your respective part of the drill: one attacks and the other defends. After you become confident in the technique, begin to add additional *retzev* counterattacks using everything you have learned. Both of you should stand in left outlet stances except for the first two drills, where the opponents stand in passive outlet stances (for practice purposes only). Practice 15 repetitions of:

1. Inside sliding parry against a straight right punch while stepping off the line

2. Inside sliding parry against a straight left punch while stepping off the line

3. Inside cross parry against a straight right punch while stepping off the line

4. Inside cross parry against a straight left punch while stepping off the line

5. Inside cross parry against a straight left/right punch combination

6. Two-handed sliding block against straight right punch with right knee attack while stepping off the line to the left

7. Two-handed sliding block against straight left punch

with left knee attack while stepping off the line to the right

8. Outside body defense with straight punch to split attacker's hands
9. Deflect and scoop defense against left/right combination
10. Trap against opponent's lead arm with over-the-top elbow strike or straight punch to the throat
11. Outside defenses against straight punches

Lower-Body Combatives

These drills focus on specific lower body combatives from chapter 3. Hold the pad straight and stand firm to absorb the power behind each of these lower-body combatives, practicing 15 repetitions of:

1. Half-roundhouse knee
2. Stepping sidekick
3. Spinning sidekick
4. Upper-body trap with offensive knee against attacker standing in left outlet stance

Kick/Knee Strikes and Combination Pad Work

To complete these drills, you will need a sturdy kicking pad. Practice your kicks and knees, driving through the pad. Be careful not to hyperextend your knee or twist your ankle.

Kick/Knee Defense Drills

Your partner kicks as you defend against the kick. Partners should kick with control and accuracy to ensure safety and allow the drill to function properly. Shin guards are recommended. Over time you may wish to discard them and condition your legs to increasingly stronger levels of impact. Practice 15 repetitions of:

1. Instinctive inside deflection with palm heel/forearm
2. Scoop defenses using inside and outside hooks against straight kicks and sidekicks
3. Inside deflection against a high straight kick to the head
4. Sliding deflection defense against straight kick from the rear
5. Body defense moving off the line

Timing Drills

Timing drills develop your self-defense capabilities and fighting prowess. For these drills, you will work slowly with your partner. As your partner delivers a punch or kick, you will move away, out of the kick's reach, and then follow up with your own punch or kick.

Your Twelve-Week Program

Practice the following drills, many of which you may already be familiar with, three to four times a week, with a day of rest between workouts. Combine the upper-body combative drills in the first column, lower-body combative drills in the second column, and the combination drills in the third column into one comprehensive workout. Each week, your *krav maga* workout will become somewhat longer and more intense as you build your skills and fitness. This program incorporates most of the techniques from the preceding chapters, many of which you refamiliarized yourself with at the beginning of this chapter. While not emphasized in the following *kravist* workouts, releases from chapter 5 can be incorporated at the end of the workout. The following techniques and combinations, first practiced in repetition and then combined into *retzev*, provide a rigorous cardiovascular and muscular workout for your entire body.

Schedule	Upper-Body Combative Drills	Lower-Body Combative Drills	Upper-Body & Lower-Body Combinations
WEEK 1 Use proper footwork to move in and out with combinations. You may also close your eyes to perform combinations by envisioning boxing movements. For lateral movements (from the left outlet stance), draw your right foot back to break the angle followed by the left foot. Do the opposite movements from a right outlet stance.	SOLO From the left outlet stance: • 15 repetitions of the front straight punch (review) • 15 repetitions of the rear straight punch (review) • 15 repetitions of the front half-roundhouse punch • 15 repetitions of the rear half-roundhouse punch • 15 repetitions of the straight front/rear and front/rear half-roundhouse punch combinations with step and pivot • Repeat each drill from the right outlet stance, reversing the movements accordingly WITH A PARTNER • 15 repetitions of the inside sliding parry defense against a straight right punch while stepping off the line • 15 repetitions of the inside sliding parry defense against a straight left punch while stepping off the line into collar or triangle chokes	SOLO From the left outlet stance: • 15 repetitions of the front half-roundhouse knee • 15 repetitions of the rear half-roundhouse knee • 15 repetitions of the rear half-roundhouse knee combination by alternating legs with proper pivoting using the rear leg to step forward—you are alternating each side • Repeat each drill from the right outlet stance, reversing the movements accordingly WITH A PARTNER • 15 repetitions defending against a straight kick using the instinctive inside deflection with palm heel and counterattacks Partner pad work: • 15 repetitions of the front and rear half-roundhouse knee with each leg with proper *glicha* slide step and pivot • 15 repetitions of the rear half-roundhouse knee	SOLO From the left outlet stance: • 15 repetitions of the straight left/right punch followed by 15 repetitions of the left/right half-roundhouse punch with forward movement followed by *retzev* • 15 repetitions of the front left half-roundhouse knee with forward movement followed by a left straight punch followed by *retzev.* • 15 repetitions of the rear right half-rear roundhouse knee with forward movement and right straight punch followed by a left straight punch followed by *retzev* • Repeat each drill from the right outlet stance, reversing the movements accordingly • Repeat the same drills adding a rear half-roundhouse knee followed by a forward roundhouse knee 3 minutes of *retzev* using punch variations, knees, and kicks from week 1

Schedule	Upper-Body Combative Drills	Lower-Body Combative Drills	Upper-Body & Lower-Body Combinations
WEEK 1	SOLO Partner pad work: • 15 repetitions of the straight front/rear punch combination followed by front/rear half-round-house punch combination with proper pivoting	SOLO combination by alternating legs with proper pivoting using the rear leg to step forward—you are alternating each side	SOLO
WEEK 2	SOLO • Repeat week 1 using 5 repetitions for each punch and punch combination from both outlet stances From the left outlet stance: • 15 repetitions of the straight front forearm strike • 15 repetitions of the rear forearm strike •10 repetitions of the front/rear forearm strike combination with proper pivoting and hip movement • Repeat each drill from the right outlet stance reversing the movements accordingly Upper-body combination drill: *Cont'd*	SOLO • Repeat week 1 using 10 repetitions for each kick from both outlet stances From the left outlet stance: • 15 repetitions of the stepping side kick • 15 repetitions of the stepping side kick into a sweep using the opposite leg • Repeat the drill from the right outlet stance, reversing the movements accordingly WITH A PARTNER • 15 scoop defense repetitions against the straight kick using inside deflection and *Cont'd*	SOLO • Repeat week 1 using 10 repetitions for each knee/punch combination from both outlet stances followed by a stepping side kick 4 minutes of *retzev* using different variations and combinations of punch, elbows, knees, and kicks from week 1

Schedule	Upper-Body Combative Drills	Lower-Body Combative Drills	Upper-Body & Lower-Body Combinations
WEEK 2	SOLO • 10 repetitions of the front/rear half-roundhouse punch followed by the front/rear half forearm strike • Repeat each drill from the right outlet stance	SOLO outside hooks (remember, your partner must deliver proper straight kicks by pivoting on the ball of the base leg foot and turning the base leg 90 degrees to allow for full extension of the hip and maximum reach) • Repeat the scoop defense drill against side kicks Partner pad work: • 15 repetitions of the stepping side kick to drive through the pad	SOLO
WEEK 3	SOLO • Repeat weeks 1–2 using 4 repetitions for each punch and punch combination from both outlet stances From the left outlet stance: • 15 repetitions of the front web strike to the throat • 15 repetitions of the rear web strike to the throat • 10 repetitions of the front/rear web strike to the throat	SOLO • Repeat weeks 1–2 using 4 repetitions for each kick and kick combination from both outlet stances From the left outlet stance: • 15 repeti-tions of the spinning side kick with the rear leg with a proper spin by the head leading the body • Repeat each drill from the right outlet stance, reversing	SOLO Repeat weeks 1–2 using 4 repetitions • 15 repetitions of the stepping side kick, followed by a spinning side kick using the other leg. • 5 repetitions of the side kick extension and balance drill for each leg. One partner should clasp his nearside hand with the other partner and then position himself in the initial stage of the kick with his leg cocked and heel

Schedule	Upper-Body Combative Drills	Lower-Body Combative Drills	Upper-Body & Lower-Body Combinations
WEEK 3	SOLO combination with proper pivoting • Repeat each drill from the right outlet stance Upper-body combination drill • 10 repetitions of the left front half-roundhouse punch followed by a right web strike to the throat combination with proper pivoting. Repeat the drill from the right outlet stance • Perform the same web-strike drills but alternate the web strike and half-roundhouse punch, inter-changing the front and rear arms • The front/rear roundhouse punch combi-nation at the same level and then alternate high and low punches with opposite arms WITH A PARTNER Partner pad work: • Repeat the above combi-nation half-roundhouse/web strike punch with a hand pad (be sure the pad is *Cont'd*	SOLO the movements accordingly WITH A PARTNER • 15 repetitions of the inside L deflection against a high straight kick to the head • Repeat the drill from the right outlet stance, reversing the movements accordingly	SOLO resting against the other partner's midsection. Once in position the partner positioned to side-kick will extend his leg against the partner, creating separation between them. The partner absorbing the simulated push kick should offer moderate resis-tance. Perform the drill on both legs with each partner taking turns. If properly done, this will enhance your form and balance, with your partner also learning absorption to toughen the body. • 5 minutes of *retzev* using punches, elbows, knees, and kicks and the stepping side kick/outside chop combination along with additional combatives from week 3

Schedule	Upper-Body Combative Drills	Lower-Body Combative Drills	Upper-Body & Lower-Body Combinations
WEEK 3	SOLO turned to the side for striking partner to hit the edge, taking great care not to injure the thumb); after the web strike the partner will rotate the pad to the striking partner for the powerful half-roundhouse punch combination	SOLO	SOLO
WEEK 4	SOLO • Repeat weeks 1–3 using 4 repetitions for each punch and punch combination from both outlet stances From the left outlet stance: • 15 repetitions of the rear high forearm blade across the throat • Repeat the drill from the right outlet stance, reversing the movements accordingly WITH A PARTNER • 15 repetitions of theinside L deflection against a straight right punch while stepping off the line	SOLO • Repeat weeks 1–3 using 4 repetitions for each kick and kick combination from both outlet stances WITH A PARTNER • 15 repetitions of the offensive knee and trap against attacker standing in left outlet • 15 repetitions of the sliding deflection defense against straight kick from the rear Partner pad work: • Combination kicks using straight, round-house, side, and rear defensive kicks	SOLO • Repeat weeks 1–3 using 4 repetitions for each punch and kick combination from both outlet stances • 6 minutes of *retzev* using punches, elbows, knees, and kicks in all directions from weeks 1–4 From the left outlet stance: • 15 repetitions of the straight kick with the front leg using the forward leg shuffle to step and punch with same side arm, followed by a rear straight punch, a forward horizontal elbow, a rear horizontal elbow, and a rear knee • Repeat the drill

Schedule	Upper-Body Combative Drills	Lower-Body Combative Drills	Upper-Body & Lower-Body Combinations
WEEK 4	SOLO • 15 repetitions of the inside L deflection against a straight left punch while stepping off the line Partner pad work: • 15 repetitions using clothesline forearm blade strike across the throat with striking partner stepping to the side of the target while keeping a slight bend in the elbow to prevent hyperextension (*if you do not bend the elbow you will injure yourself*) From the left outlet stance: • 15 repetitions of front arm whipping strikes to the eyes • 15 repetitions of rear arm whipping strikes to the eyes • 10 repetitions of the combination front whipping strike to the eye followed by the rear web strike to the throat • Repeat each drill from the right outlet stance	SOLO	SOLO from the left outlet stance • 7 minutes of *retzev* using punches, elbows, knees, and kicks in all directions from weeks 1–5 WITH A PARTNER • 5-minute drill of partners using timing to exchange kicks (including: half-roundhouse knee, stepping sidekick, and spinning sidekick) without contact. One partner follows through with a kick while the other partner retreats using a body defense and then delivers his own kick. In short, partners will trade kicks with no contact. As one partner withdraws his kick, the other partner initiates his. Precision, control, and timing are the focus.

Schedule	Upper-Body Combative Drills	Lower-Body Combative Drills	Upper-Body & Lower-Body Combinations
WEEK 4	SOLO WITH A PARTNER • 15 repetitions of the two-handed sliding block against straight right punch with right knee attack while stepping off the line to the left • 15 repetitions of the two-handed sliding block against straight left punch with left knee attack while stepping off the line to the right	SOLO	SOLO
WEEK 5	SOLO • Repeat weeks 1–4 using 4 repetitions for each punch and punch combination from both outlet stances. From the left outlet stance: • 15 repetitions of the over-the-top punch, making sure your striking arm moves high to low • 15 repetitions of the knuckle edge strike to the throat • Repeat each drill from the right outlet stance	SOLO • Repeat weeks 1–4 using 4 repetitions for each kick and kick combination from both outlet stances WITH A PARTNER • 15 repetitions of the instinctive inside deflection with palm heel/forearm retreat against a straight kick	SOLO • Repeat weeks 1–4 using 4 repetitions for each punch and kick combination from both outlet stances WITH A PARTNER • Partners use timing to exchange knees and stepping and spinning side kicks using forward and retreating movements. This drill differs from week 4's workout because you and your partner are moving in and out without contact for five minutes.

Schedule	Upper-Body Combative Drills	Lower-Body Combative Drills	Upper-Body & Lower-Body Combinations
WEEK 5	SOLO WITH A PARTNER • 15 repetitions of left/right straight punch deflection and angled gunt	SOLO	SOLO One partner follows through with a kick while the other partner retreats using a body defense and then delivers his own kick. In short, partners will trade kicks with no contact. As one partner is withdrawing his kick, the other partner initiates his. Precision, control, and timing are the focus. You may add additional kicks that you know to the drill as well. • 15 repetitions of the roundhouse kick with the front leg, followed by a straight front arm punch, followed by a straight rear arm punch, followed by a rear roundhouse kick. Strive to create seamless movement and flow between your hands and feet. • Repeat each drill from the right outlet stance • 8 minutes of *retzev* using punches, elbows, knees, and kicks in all directions Partner pad work: *Cont'd*

Schedule	Upper-Body Combative Drills	Lower-Body Combative Drills	Upper-Body & Lower-Body Combinations
WEEK 5	SOLO	SOLO	SOLO • One partner holds a shield and feigns a punching motion. The other partner knees the shield with a half-roundhouse knee (using control) with his hands up to defend the punch. This is not a power-centric drill. Remember the partner holding the shield is extending himself to punch, making the body vulnerable behind the shield. This drill simulates a timing kick to preempt an incoming straight or hook punch. I often have students use a foam stick to simulate the reach of a punch to help perfect timing. • One partner holds a hand pad (away from the face) and feigns a hook punch. The defending partner uses timing to deliver a straight punch to the pad. This drill simulates a direct strike to block a circular or looping type of attack.

Schedule	Upper-Body Combative Drills	Lower-Body Combative Drills	Upper-Body & Lower-Body Combinations
WEEK 6	SOLO • Repeat weeks 1–5 using 5 repetitions for each punch and punch combination from both outlet stances • 15 repetitions of parry and trap with immediate counterpunch against the straight left/right punch combination WITH A PARTNER • 15 repetitions of the inward chop • 15 repetitions of the outward chop Combinations: • 15 repetitions of the double chop, using a front chop followed instantaneously with a rear chop to the same target	SOLO • Repeat weeks 1–5 using 5 repetitions for each kick and kick combination from both outlet stances WITH A PARTNER From the left outlet stance: • 15 repetitions of scoop defenses using inside and outside hook deflections against the straight kick • 15 repetitions of inside deflection against high kick	SOLO • Repeat weeks 1–5 using 5 repetitions for each kick and kick combination from both outlet stances. Try combining all these drills, adding two additional combatives, then four additional combatives, then six additional combatives, and so on to build your *retzev*. • 9 minutes of *retzev* using punches, elbows, knees, and kicks in all directions from weeks 1–6
WEEK 7	SOLO Repeat weeks 1–6, using 3 repetitions for each punch and punch combination from both outlet stances WITH A PARTNER *Cont'd*	SOLO Repeat weeks 1–6, using 3 repetitions for each kick and kick combination from both outlet stances. WITH A PARTNER *Cont'd*	SOLO Repeat weeks 1–6, using 3 repetitions for each kick and kick combination from both outlet stances. Combine all these drills, adding two additional combatives, then four additional *Cont'd*

Schedule	Upper-Body Combative Drills	Lower-Body Combative Drills	Upper-Body & Lower-Body Combinations
WEEK 7	SOLO • 15 repetitions of inside sliding parry against a straight right punch while stepping off the line • 15 repetitions of inside sliding parry against a straight left punch while stepping off the line	SOLO From the left outlet stance: • 15 repetitions of sliding deflection defense against front and rear straight kicks • 15 repetitions of body defense and counterattack against a straight kick by moving off the line	SOLO combatives, then six additional combatives, and so on. 10 minutes of *retzev* using punches, elbows, knees, and kicks in all directions
WEEK 8	SOLO • Repeat weeks 1–7, using 3 repetitions for each punch and punch combination from both outlet stances WITH A PARTNER • 15 repetitions of the inside L block against a straight left punch followed by *retzev* combatives, then repeat the drill against a right punch; switch your stance from left outlet to right outlet and perform the drill again WITH A PARTNER • 15 repetitions of the parallel	SOLO • Repeat weeks 1–7, using 3 repetitions for each kick and kick combination from both outlet stances with a partner From the left outlet stance: • Sliding deflection defense against side kick From the left outlet stance: • High round-house kick defenses using a parallel gunt and inside movement to close the distance with simultaneous counterattack • 15 repetitions of defense against high roundhouse	SOLO • 11 minutes of *retzev* using punches, elbows, knees, and kicks in all directions Repeat weeks 1–7, using 3 repetitions for each kick and kick combination from both outlet stances WITH A PARTNER • From the left outlet stance, the defender traps the attacker's arms (also standing in an outlet stance) inwards and executes offensive knee with proper pivot pulling attacker's arms to generate additional momentum For defenses against combinations, mentally visualize the defenses you

Schedule	Upper-Body Combative Drills	Lower-Body Combative Drills	Upper-Body & Lower-Body Combinations

WEEK 8	SOLO
	
	gunt against a hook punch
	
	• 15 repetitions of the trap against opponent's lead arm with an over-the-top elbow strike to the temple or over-the-top punch to the throat
		SOLO
		
		kick double arm deflection
		
		WITH A PARTNER
		
		• 15 repetitions of defenses against the high side kick to the head
		• 15 repetitions of outside vertical gunt against a high roundhouse kick
		• 15 repetitions of late defense against low roundhouse kick
		• 15 repetitions of the following defenses against sweeps using each defense you have learned:
		    –Body defense and pick up front leg
		    –Defensive kick (front/back) to body
		    –Close the distance with hand attacks (timing)
		    –Change legs (rear leg) to avoid sweep
		• 15 repetitions of feinting the straight kick into roundhouse kick using either leg
		• Straight kick feint into side kick using the rear leg
			SOLO
			
			would use against all of the combinations you have learned. Two examples might include:
			• Defend against a straight kick to groin and punch to the face (inside deflections and counterattacks)
			• Defend against a roundhouse kick at varying heights and punches that may be used in combination following the kick
			• 12 minutes of *retzev* using punches, elbows, knees, and kicks in all directions
			
			WITH A PARTNER
			
			• From the outlet stance, the defender splits the attacker's arms (also standing in an outlet stance), using a wedge motion by placing the palms together and diving inward while executing the offensive knee
			• Body absorption drill: partner works at moving with strikes and absorbing blows while exhaling (the drill can also be performed with the eyes closed-but partners must observe careful control of strikes)

WEEK 9

WITH A PARTNER

CLINCHES
Practice each of these clinch unbalancing positional exercises for 3 minutes apiece:
1. Crown-of-the-head clinch
2. Symmetrical clinch
3. Crown-of-the-head cant clinch into *tsai-bake* into takedown

TAKEDOWNS AND CONTROL
15 repetitions of:
1. Cavalier
2. Shirt-grab defenses
3. Control hold 1
4. Control hold 2
5. Bucket-scoop takedown
6. Double leg takedown tackle
7. Double leg takedown tackle boxing defense

Complete 12 minutes of standing *retzev*

WEEK 10

WITH A PARTNER

GROUNDWORK BODY POSITIONING DRILL
Practice this drill for 3 minutes: one training partner lies flat with hands at the side while the other training partner plants his chest on the other training partner's to begin familiarizing both training partners with ground positioning; the training partner on top will use the palms of his hands and balls of the feet to perform a 360-degree circle with his weight bearing down on the training partner's chest.

OFFENSES FROM THE REAR MOUNT
Chokes
Perform 10 repetitions with each arm and simulated heel strikes to the groin:
1. Blade of the forearm
2. Crook of the elbow
3. Professional choke hold
4. Face bar

ATTACKS FROM THE BACK
Perform 10 repetitions from each side (where applicable):
1. Defense against the training partner attempting a rear mount when you are on all fours
2. Leg lock from behind, folding training partner's legs with weight against them, and choke

Arm bars

Perform 10 repetitions from each side:

1. Basic
2. Scissors (when training partner is trying to pull through) combined with fall
3. Breaking the angle and taking off balance when training partner attempts to stand
4. If your training partner is on the bottom and turns to the side, create the arm bar by taking opposite leg and placing in front of training partner's head, keeping elbow close; clamp legs down for added pressure
5. Scissors arm bar as your training partner attempts to stand
6. Arm bar using feint to opposite arm (if training partner performs defense by grabbing training partner's other arm, switch arms immediately and move in opposite direction)

Defenses Against the Arm Bar

Perform 5 repetitions from each side:

First defense: Turn into your training partner with your elbow tip down, putting pressure against the training partner's groin while reaching through with your other arm and clasping your hands to ensure the elbow is protected (do not allow your training partner to pincer his legs)

Second defense: Use your compression technique to force all of your weight forward, preventing the attacker form extending his hips while simultaneously putting tremendous pressure on his neck and spine

Complete 13 minutes of standing *retzev*

WEEK 11

WITH A PARTNER

OFFENSES FROM THE MOUNT

Trapping the training partner's arms for *retzev* combatives

Complete 5 minutes of ground *retzev.*

MOUNTED SHIELD DRILL

Straddle two shields and add a hand pad on top to simulate an opponent's head or use a heavy bag/punching dummy. Use various combatives including straight punches, half-roundhouse punches, vertical elbows, hammerfists and forearm strikes to simulate battering an opponent. Your training partner may wish to help hold the shields in place along with the hand pad. This drill simulates the rear mount and mount. You can also use the pads or heavy bag/punching dummy to practice a side mount and deliver withering knee strikes.

Mounted Partner Drill

You and your training partner will assume the mounted position. The mounted person will try to maintain the mount while the mountee attempts to escape using the various techniques you have learned, including bridging, trapping an arm and bridging, knee pushbacks, and other evasive drills.

Practice the following drills 5 repetitions per arm side:
1. Brace to the throat or jaw
2. Defending against brace to the throat and jaw
   Practice trapping your partner's arms and delivering combatives. Your partner may then practice defenses against traps and *retzev* combatives.

Practice 10 repetitions from each side where applicable:
1. The side ground headlock chest up
2. Release against side ground headlock
3. Release against side ground headlock variation

Transition from the guard to the mount and do 3 repetitions of week 10
Complete 14 minutes of standing *retzev*

WEEK 12

Review and repeat 2 repetitions of each drill from weeks 10 and 11

WITH A PARTNER

OFFENSES FROM SIDE MOUNT POSITION
Practice 10 repetitions from each side where applicable:
1. Knee combatives chest down
2. Baby pressure triangular choke and cervical pressure holds from side control chest down

Have a training partner hold two kicking shields on the ground. You may want to add a hand pad for a facsimile head. You may also use a heavy bag to simulate an opponent. Practice each of these drills for four 3-minute intervals:

Sidemount Drill
   Simulate your side control position by resting your body weight on the pads while on the balls of your feet. Deliver straight and roundhouse knees in rapid succession. Be sure your training partner is well anchored behind the pads to absorb the tremendous force you will generate. Try to turn the base leg as you deliver the knee—as with our standing knees, this will generate the most power.

Knee-on-Stomach Drill
   Simulate your knee-on-the-stomach position by resting your knee and entire body weight on the pads while on the ball of your rear foot and flat of your front foot with approximately a 45-degree bend in the knee. Deliver straight punches in rapid succession against the pad. Be sure your training partner is well anchored behind the pads to absorb the tremendous force you will generate. Try to turn the base leg as you deliver the knee—as with our standing knees, this will generate the most power.

Practice 10 repetitions from each side where applicable:
4. The side ground headlock chest up
5. Release against side ground headlock
6. Release against side ground headlock variation

Transition from the guard to the mount and repeat 3 repetitions of week 10

GUARD WORK

Offenses from the High Closed Guard
Practice 10 repetitions from each side with your partner in your guard:
1. Arm bar transition from the high closed guard
2. Triangular leg choke with combatives from your back and side
3. Front ground headlock choke or guillotine
4. Arm bar by sliding legs up and across the face or behind the neck into the arm bar
5. Defenses against Achilles leg lock and ankle locks

Defenses Against the Guard and Triangle Choke
Practice 10 repetitions against your partner's closed guard:
1. Maintaining posture and delivering groin strikes
2. Basic release against the triangular leg choke
3. Leg and ankle locks
4. Vertical stacking
5. Release against front guillotine choke

Complete 15 minutes of standing *retzev*

Twelve Weeks and Beyond

Once you have completed the twelve-week program, continue to practice *krav maga*, using the drills from the program as a practice guide. Combine those drills with the previous sample workouts and drills, which will help you to take your *krav maga* training to the next level.

APPENDIX

Interviews

AL BLITSTEIN

Al Blitstein, a decorated World War II veteran who served in the U.S. First and Third Armies under Generals Bradley and Patton, was a close personal friend of *krav maga* founder Imi Lichtenfeld. Al is the father of Rick Blitstein, my very good friend and first *krav maga* instructor and one of the original instructors trained directly under Imi to introduce *krav maga* to the United States. Al knew Imi for more than twenty years and visited Imi in Israel. I interviewed Al for his perspective on the early days of *krav maga* in the United States and his personal remembrances of Imi.

How did you first learn of Israeli krav maga?

I learned of Israeli *krav maga* in 1979 when Imi and some of his senior students visited Cleveland on their *krav maga* publicity tour across the United States. Rick had studied various martial arts and we decided to see what this man had to offer. We arrived early at Imi's demonstration. Rick sat at the side of the hallway. Suddenly, these imposing men came in with their white *gi* uniforms and black belts. These were tough-looking guys. When Imi saw us, he stopped and looked at Rick. Imi grabbed Rick by the hair and hoisted him and said, "Follow me." It was a strange episode for a father to see another man grabbing his son by the hair and pulling him away. What I did not realize was that Imi knew Rick already; they had met previously in Israel in 1977 on a kibbutz. Imi led just the two of us into the demonstration room. What we saw amazed us. I had never seen a group of people move like that. I asked Imi, "But what if someone had a gun in his hand?" using my pointer and thumb to simulate a gun. Imi answered my question by saying, "I would think about it and then do this." He suddenly took his hand out of his pocket and threw the coins into my face. Imi finished his thought: "While you are distracted we would move and finish you." We spent the next fifteen minutes asking about different scenarios and how they would react. I was so impressed and Rick was too, but Rick had seen some of this before. After having lived in Israel from 1976 to 1978, when he first met Imi, Rick decided to return to Israel on the personal invitation of Imi in 1981 to attend the first international instructor's course.

What do you remember from Rick about his first impressions of krav maga *training*?

Rick's first impressions were that the training was harder than he thought it would be. Rick and his fellow trainees looked forward to the training. They knew it would not be easy and it would be worth it; they would learn something very valuable. Rick earned the certificate of instructor completion signed by Imi himself. Imi said he would come to visit Rick and he did visit us. Alan Feldman, who also completed the course, and Rick were strictly Imi's students. Imi was the boss. He told them to throw a punch and he meant it. There was nothing phony ever about what Imi asked.

What did you think the first time Rick came back from Israel after his instructor training to demonstrate and teach the krav maga *he had learned from Imi*?

The first time Rick came back, he orchestrated a public demonstration. A number of people attended. He worked with his partner, Scott Black, who attended the Israeli Krav Maga Association's first international instructor course with Rick. Scott was a silver-medalist power lifter. When Scott put Rick into a headlock, Rick took Scott down so fast that Scott's body slapped the ground with a loud sound. Rick winded him with one drop. I thought, "Wow, they don't fool around." Little by little Rick and Scott showed about a dozen moves. The public was very fascinated by what they saw. Imi's legacy lives on.

What were your initial impressions of Imi when you first met him?

In the first demonstration I saw, I noticed Imi had a twisted face. I learned that Imi sustained serious injuries after he went overboard to save the *Pentcho*, bound for Palestine, by freeing its propellers. These terrible wounds he received while freeing the propellers disfigured his face. He leapt overboard because the people on board needed to make it to Israel. Their lives depended on it. As a result, he cleared the propeller. Imi was a true hero.

If you saw Imi coming toward you, you would be happy to get out of his way. The look on his face, you had to pay him respect. He always looked you directly in the eyes. He had a piercing look. He sized you up immediately. I could see he was thinking tactically. No matter what Imi did, people were impressed. Imi thought of all his students as his children. He would show his devotion directly using one or two words; no long explanations. I can say this—if Imi directed his students to get you, you would be the target of the damned toughest people you would ever have met. Imi was definitely their mentor and instructor.

Later, when I had a chance to film Imi, it was just as much fun. One memory stands out particularly. Imi had an ascot tie in his hand. With the ascot in front of him, he fashioned a noose with just one hand. He explained, "If you must have a noose to choke someone, you can make a noose that fast. No one will know what you are doing." Imi told me to make one. On the third try, I did it. I could not believe it. Imi smiled and gave me his nod of approval. Imi could teach you something without your knowing it. Imi had the appearance of a smooth talker, debonair; he was a great dancer. He had old-world charm. I felt very close to Imi and lucky to be so.

You visited with Imi in Israel?

I went to Israel, to Netanya, to visit Imi in 1985. When I arrived at the café early, Imi's students checked me out closely and followed me. When Imi saw me and greeted me, his security personnel slipped away. I sat down with Imi and told Imi that he was responsible for saving Rick's life. Imi was both relieved and alarmed. Here is the story. One day in Cleveland, Rick got out of his car and closed the door. A drunk driver was speeding down the street, nearly scraping the parked cars. Rick was in his line of fire. Rick had to think what to do to save himself. Rick jumped up into the air and landed on the top of the car with a back roll. I told Imi, "You taught him not only to move right and left but to move up or down as necessary. If you had not taught him that move, he would not be here today."

What is your favorite Imi story?

During my 1985 visit with Imi in Netanya, my wife walked away to do some window shopping. Next to his office building, there was a table set back in seclusion. Imi asked, "Where is your wife?" I said I didn't know. Imi said, "Is she there or not?" Imi immediately got up to search for her personally. To his relief, he saw her window shopping. Imi knew when to look; he was always alert. You never knew exactly what he was thinking, but you knew he was thinking about safety. Here is another one. During a demonstration with Rick and Alan in Cleveland in 1984, I asked Imi how old he was. Imi answered that he was seventy-six years old, and the audience gasped. He moved like an acrobat; you could see he was still an active man. Imi responded, "You don't have to applaud me. I know I am good."

How did krav maga *change your son's life?*

Krav maga made all the difference in Rick's life. It was like a marriage. He dedicated himself. He could not have been more changed. Rick became more studious and serious. It became part of his lifestyle. It made him a better man and a more dedicated person. Rick always found a certain humor in Imi's thinking. For example, when asked if you could continue kicking a man after you had incapacitated him. Imi's quick response that made Rick laugh was, "Why would you kick a dead man?"

RICK BLITSTEIN AND ALAN FELDMAN, TWO OF THE FIRST INTERNATIONAL *KRAV MAGA* INSTRUCTORS

I conducted separate interviews with senior instructors Rick Blitstein and Alan Feldman, two of the first Americans to complete the Israeli Krav Maga Association's international instructor's course in 1981. I asked them what it was like to become an instructor in the earliest days of *krav maga*'s growing international popularity.

Q: How did you first learn of krav maga*?*

Rick Blitstein: I was living on Kibbutz Ein Harod Me-Uchad in 1977. I had grown up learning kung fu and practiced outside on the kibbutz. Some of the *kibbutzniks* were watching and approached me. Basically, they humiliated me and beat me to a pulp, but they were seemingly impressed that I kept getting up and asking, "How did you do that?"

Alan Feldman: I read a small article in the *Jewish Exponent* in 1980 stating that *krav maga* was the hand-to-hand combat system of the Israel Defense Forces. I was definitely interested because I had studied martial arts since I was eleven years old.

Q: When did you first meet Imi?

RB: In 1977, when my commando friends took me to train and there were some older men watching. One of those men was Imi.

AF: I met Imi the first day of the 1981 international instructor's course.

Q: What were your first impressions of Imi?

RB: My first impression of Imi was that he was a man of respect. He was thoroughly a European gentleman. You could not help noticing that everyone around him respected him and that in a very simple way he earned your respect. Imi asked me in a mixture of Hebrew and Yiddish about my family background. He then asked me if I would like to learn *krav maga* in Israel. Imi invited me personally to the learn *krav maga* under his guidance. In 1979, I met Imi again in Cleveland.

AF: Ten minutes after the start of our course, Imi walked into the room impeccably dressed. Imi moved with a fluidity I had never seen.

Q: What was the first Israeli Krav Maga Association international instructor's course in 1981 like?

RB: Imi invited me personally to a future instructor's course after his visit to Cleveland in 1979. The 1981 group met at Kennedy Airport. We were picked up by a bus at Ben Gurion, which took us to the Green Beach Hotel in Netanya. We were taken to Eli Avikzar's school to watch the top Israelis in action. Their level of expertise was just amazing.

AF: It was absolutely grueling for those who were willing to work hard. We had the equivalent of four and a half years of training compressed into six weeks. Out of twenty students, only four passed with green belt instructor status. Rick and I were two of them.

Q: What was the first day of the course like?

RB: Everyone was called out individually—this was before anyone ever thought of bringing protective equipment—to be tested by two of the top Israeli instructors. We were invited to free-spar, and they made a bruising point that we had a lot to learn. We trained a minimum of six hours a day, six days a week, for the six-week course.

AF: Imi rolled up his sleeves and had one of his instructors try to stab him in the throat with a knife. After performing the defense with astounding fluidity, Imi turned to us and stated, "Look who gets the punch." I leaned back and thought, "Why didn't I think of that after thirteen years of martial arts training?" I was hooked.

Q: Was the course more difficult or less difficult than you antici-pated?

RB: The course was much more difficult. The course was grueling because there was very little time to heal. Not only did the Israelis beat us up, but we were forced to beat the hell out of each other.

AF: To me, the course was hard as hell, but I would not characterize it as difficult, just hard as hell. In fact, I was so addicted that after our course ended, occasionally we went to other instructors' schools.

Q: Did you make lasting friends from the course?

RB: One friend, Alan—who split my forehead.

AF: Rick and I gravitated to each other from the start.

Q: What is your favorite Imi story?

RB: There are so many, but one time in particular stands out. Imi was a professional ballroom dancer and an accomplished hummer. He danced with women by humming a waltz.

AF: My favorite Imi story was sitting in my apartment with Imi and Rick. We were watching *Return of the Dragon* featuring Bruce Lee and Chuck Norris. In the Colosseum fight Bruce Lee ducked under Chuck Norris's kick. Imi quickly said, "I know the boy is good, but if he can duck he can go inside." I said to Imi, "Yes, that makes sense, but then the fight would be over and no more movie!" I also note a story which Rick also witnessed in Café Oogahtee in Netanya. A man in his eighties leaned over to us and said, "Let me tell you how Imi fought. Imi only delivered one punch; one punch would end the man." Imi confirmed this story when telling us of the many times he had to put his back against the wall when outnumbered.

Q: What is your favorite saying of Imi's?

RB: "The leg of a baby is stronger than the balls of Muhammad Ali."

AF: "You must learn to be so good that you don't have to kill." But I can't just choose one: "Everybody respects strength" and "You offer peace from a position of strength."

Q: What is the most important aspect to keep in mind for those who would like to train in krav maga?

RB: To respect your training partner and to not hurt each other. *Krav maga* is not a sport. People can seriously hurt each other if training improperly.

AF: Empty your cup. Approach *krav maga* with an open mind. Each aspect of the system is based on reality. Simplify your movements and leave the complicated stuff behind.

Q: What is the most important aspect to keep in mind for those who would like to teach krav maga?

RB: To realize this is not a game. Never forget the purpose of training and where *krav maga* comes from.

AF: The student must leave with a higher level of confidence than when he came in. One of the most important aspects of *krav maga* instruction is instilling confidence. Most important, there must be safety in training.

Q: Why do you think krav maga has become so popular all over the world?

RB: Imi's genius accounts for its popularity. The Israeli Krav Maga Association continues Imi's legacy. *Krav maga* is simple to learn for anyone regardless of stature, gender, nationality, or age. Also, unfortunately, there is a need and demand for it all over the world.

AF: In 1984, Imi was visiting me in Philadelphia and predicted, "Soon, everyone will come to our way of thinking." In my opinion, any fight training gravitates to the practical. Also, despite many difficulties, I would hope the majority of *krav maga* schools can find common ground and think of themselves as family.

RESOURCES

For protective padding and other supplies:

Asian World of Martial Arts
9400 Ashton Road
Philadelphia, PA 19114
1-800-345-2962
www.awma.com

Aries Fight Gear
Aries Sports Industries, Inc.
1838 Route 7A
P.O. Box 195
Shaftsbury, VT 08562
1-800-542-7437
www.ariesfightgear.com

Israel Military Products
P.O. Box 31006
Tel Aviv 61310
Israel
In United States: 1-888-293-1421 or 1-718-701-3955

In Israel: 972-3-6204612; fax 972-9-8859661

www.israelmilitary.com

To read more about *krav maga* and its history:

The Israel Defense Forces
www.idf.il
The Israeli Special Forces
www.isayeret.com
The International Defense Force
www.i-d-f.com

ABOUT THE AUTHOR

David Kahn, United States Chief instructor for the Israeli Krav Maga, received his advanced black-belt teaching certifications from Grandmaster Haim Gidon and is the only American to sit on the Israeli Krav Maga Association's board of directors. David trains regularly in Israel and holds the distinction of having trained in Israel more than any American instructor. David is committed to the proper expansion of the Israeli *krav maga* system in the United States and worldwide. David has been featured in *Men's Fitness*, *The New Yorker*, *Penthouse*, *Fitness*, *Traveler*, *Self*, *Allure*, *The Los Angeles Times*, *The Washington Post*, and a host of other publications. David is certified as an instructor by the State of New Jersey Police Training Commission. Trainees include federal, state, and local law enforcement professionals, military personnel, celebrities, executives, fitness enthusiasts, and others. David, his brother, Abel, his father, Alfred, and Emmy and Golden Globe Award–winner James Gandolfini opened the Israeli Krav Maga U.S. Training Center in February 2007.

The Israeli Krav Maga U.S. Training Center serves as the IKMA's United States training hub, sponsoring full-time classes, specialty seminars, and law enforcement and military training, including Israeli-based counterterror instruction and Israeli tactical shooting along with *krav maga* instructor certification courses. Grandmaster Gidon and other top-ranking Israeli instructors regularly visit David's classes. David also has teaching programs at the David Barton Gyms, the 92nd Street Y Makor organization, the Jewish Community Center in Manhattan, and his alma mater, Princeton University. David lives in New Jersey. For more information, contact:

Israeli Krav Maga U.S. Training Center
127 Route 206, Unit 9
Hamilton, New Jersey 08610
(609) 585-MAGA
www.israelikrav.com

Israeli Krav Maga Association
P.O. Box 1103
Netanya
Israel
www.kravmagaisraeli.com